Practical Physiology
for
Dental Students

Text and Viva Voce

Questions and Answers

Highlights of this unique title:

1. Practical skills [comprehensive coverage of practicals with Objective Structured Practical Examination (OSPE) and Objective Structured Clinical Examination (OSCE) questions]

2. Multiple choice questions

3. Viva voce questions

4. Clinical case scenario for understanding the concept of applied clinical physiology in oral health

5. Historical aspects and recent advances of every topic

6. Guide for preparing for applied physiology questions of All India BDS Entrance and PG Dental Entrance Examinations of all health universities/deemed universities

7. A pocket guide for dental practitioners

Practical Physiology
for
Dental Students

Text and Viva Voce

Questions and Answers

NA John
MBBS, MD, DIH, FPGDMLE, PGDMLE (Medical Law and Ethics)

Professor and Head
Department of Physiology, and
Dean of Examination
All India Institute of Medical Sciences
Bibinagar, Hyderabad, AP

Ex-Professor and Head
Indira Gandhi Medical College and Research Institute
Puducherry

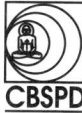

CBSPD

CBS Publishers & Distributors Pvt Ltd

New Delhi • Bengaluru • Chennai • Kochi • Kolkata • Lucknow • Mumbai
Hyderabad • Jharkhand • Nagpur • Patna • Pune • Uttarakhand

Practical Physiology
for
Dental Students

ISBN: 978-81-239-2847-0

Copyright © Author and Publisher

First Edition: 2016
Reprint: 2021, **2024**

Published by Satish Kumar Jain and produced by Varun Jain for

CBS Publishers & Distributors Pvt Ltd
4819/XI Prahlad Street, 24 Ansari Road, Daryaganj, New Delhi 110 002, India.
Ph: 011-23289259, 23266838

Website: www.cbspd.com
e-mail: delhi@cbspd.com

Corporate Office: 204 FIE, Industrial Area, Patparganj, Delhi 110 092
Ph: 011-4934 4934   Fax: 011-4934 4935   e-mail: publishing@cbspd.com;
publicity@cbspd.com

Branches

- **Bengaluru:** Seema House 2975, 17th Cross, K.R. Road, Banasankari 2nd Stage, Bengaluru 560 070, Karnataka, India
  Ph: +91-80-26771678/79   Fax: +91-80-26771680   e-mail: bangalore@cbspd.com
- **Chennai:** Subbaraya Street, Shenoy Nagar, Chennai 600 030, Tamil Nadu, India
  Ph: +91-44-26680620/26681266   Fax: +91-44-42032115   e-mail: chennai@cbspd.com
- **Kochi:** 42/1325, 1326, Power House Road, Opp KSEB, Ernakulam 682 018, Kochi, Kerala, India
  Ph: +91-484-4059061-65, 67   Fax: +91-484-4059065   e-mail: kochi@cbspd.com
- **Kolkata:** 147, Hind Ceramics Compound, 1st Floor, Nilgunj road, Belghoria, Kolkata 700056, West Bengal, India
  Ph: 033-25633055/56   e-mail: kolkata@cbspd.com
- **Lucknow:** Basement, Khushnuma Complex, 7-Meerabai Marg (Behind Jawahar Bhawan), Lucknow-226 001, Uttar Pradesh, India.
  Ph: +0552-4000032   e-mail:tiwari.lucknowi@cbspd.com
- **Mumbai:** PWD shed, Gala No. 25/26, Ramchandra Bhatt Marg, Next to JJ Hospital Gate No. 2, OPP, Union Bank of India, Noorbaug, Mumbai-400009, Maharashtra, India
  Ph: 022-66661880/89   e-mail: mumbai@cbspd.com

Representatives

- **Hyderabad** 0-9885175004
- **Patna** 0-9334159340
- **Jharkhand** 0-9811541605
- **Pune** 0-9664372571
- **Nagpur** 0-8692091830
- **Uttarakhand** 0-9716462459

Printed at: Mudrak, Noida, India

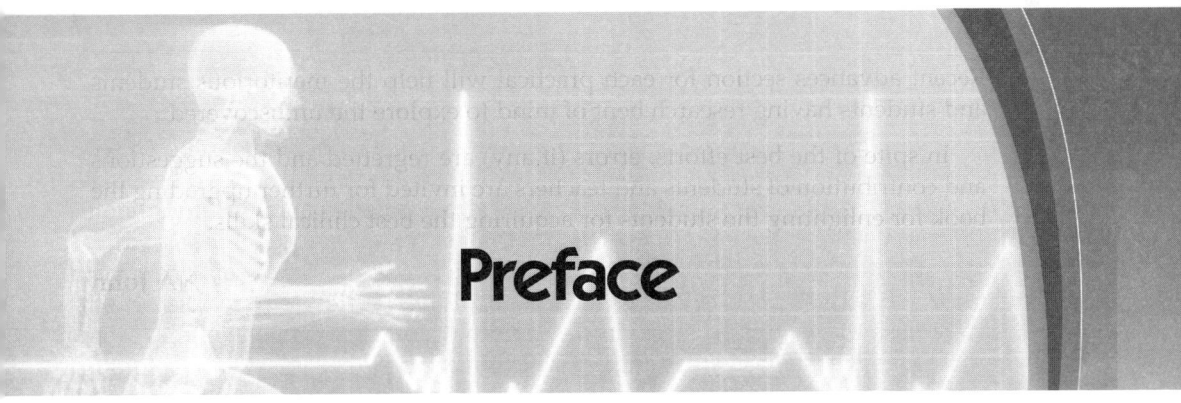

Preface

In view of scarcity of practical books in physiology centered around dental perspectives and applied clinical physiology toward dental health, the present book has been exclusively written for dental undergraduate and postgraduate students for giving them comprehensive knowledge of practical physiology based on the curriculum and syllabus designed by the Dental Council of India and various state health universities and deemed universities.

Every topic is covered with special emphasis on applied clinical physiology in oral health and diseases.

The key features of the book include:

(1) Structured objectives behind learning every practical.

(2) The procedures and explanations are crisp and to the point.

(3) Objective structured clinical examination has been covered for each practical.

(4) Historical aspects and scientific contributions in developing techniques of important practicals have been elaborated.

(5) Multiple choice questions for practical will help the student to have self-assessment regarding extent to which he/she has understood the topic. The multiple choice questions with key will be helpful for students to prepare for theory and practical examinations, viva voce and postgraduate entrance examination.

(6) Clinical case scenarios exclusively covering applied clinical physiology and its implications on oral health will help the BDS undergraduate students to have sound foundation knowledge of dental physiology and oral biology. The clinical case scenarios and MCQs will be of immense help while preparing for All India Postgraduate Dental Entrance Examination and Postgraduate Dental Entrance Examinations of various universities and deemed universities.

(7) It can be a reference guide for private dental practitioners for updating the techniques and acquiring knowledge regarding recent advances in the subject.

(8) Recent advances section for each practical will help the meritorious students and students having research bent of mind to explore the undiscovered.

In spite of the best efforts, errors (if any) are regretted and the suggestions and contribution of students and teachers are invited for further upgrading the book for enlighting the students for acquiring the best clinical skills.

NA John

Contents

Introduction

- Study of a compound microscope
- Methods of collection of blood
- Hemocytometry

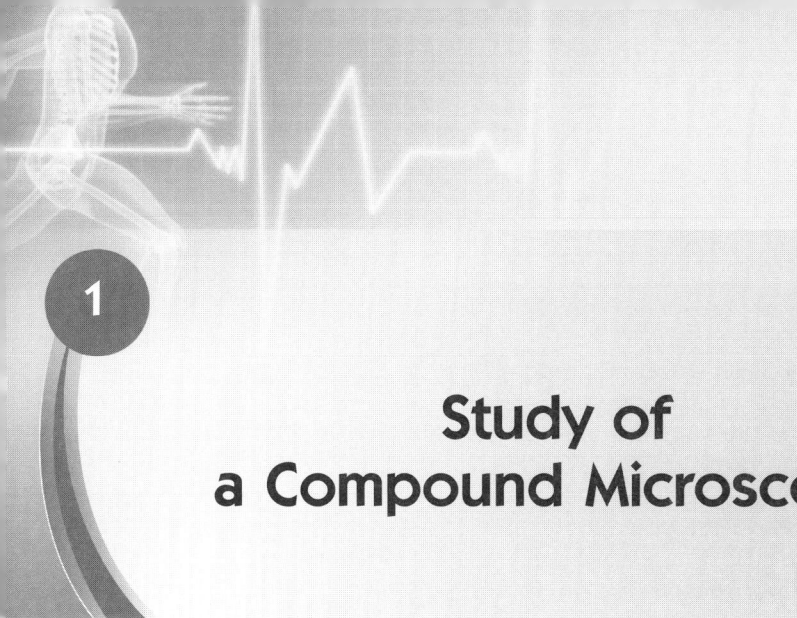

Study of a Compound Microscope

Learning Objectives

The student after doing the experiment should be able to:

1. Identify the parts of a compound microscope.
2. Focus the given blood smear using low power, high power and oil immersion objective lenses.
3. Understand the importance of learning microscopy and its implication in dental practice.

INTRODUCTION

Microscope is an instrument used to visualize objects which cannot be seen by the naked eye. Compound microscope is an instrument for magnifying small objects. It consists of an objective lens of short focal length for forming an image and that is further magnified by a second lens (eyepiece) of longer focal length. The two lenses are mounted in the same tube.

TYPES OF MICROSCOPES

Light microscope: The lenses refract light to make the object beneath them appear closer. Common magnifications: X40, X100 and X400.

Stereoscope: This microscope allows for binocular (two eyes) viewing of larger specimens.

Scanning electron microscope: It uses electrons (negatively charged electrical particles) to magnify objects up to two million times.

Transmission electron microscope: It also uses electrons, but instead of scanning the surface (as with scanning electron microscope) electrons are passed through very thin specimens.

DENTAL PERSPECTIVE

The introduction of the microscope into precision dental practice has been immensely helpful in operative dental surgery. The magnification and adequate lighting help to see better, provide better patient care and produce higher quality dentistry. The students should learn the techniques of art of careful observation and working in an appropriate ergonomic position for better visualization while learning hematology practical skills as these skills are latter useful to have further competency while using surgical microscopes as dental surgeon. The students should note that a basic surgical microscope is an optical instrument consisting of a combination of lenses which provide the surgeon with a stereoscopic, high quality magnified image of small structures within the surgical field of operation. The microscopes are designed ergonomically so that the surgeon remains comfortable and free of eyestrain.

PARTS OF THE MICROSCOPE

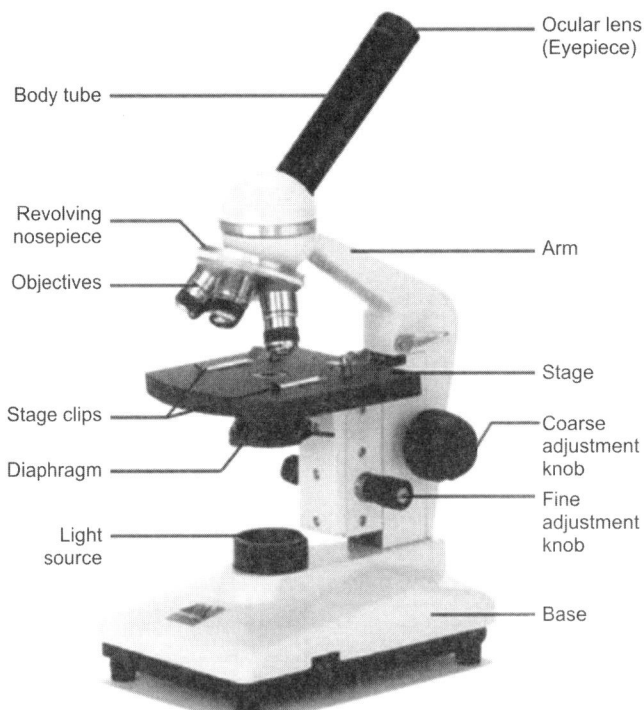

Fig. 1.1 Compound microscope

Optical System: Ocular Lens and Eyepiece

The microscope consists of an optical system of lenses and it magnifies the given object. A simple microscope has one lens while a compound microscope has more lenses.

Base: The microscope has a solid base which provides stability.

Arm: The handle supports the optical system of lenses and can be used for lifting the microscope.

Mirror: Light from an electric bulb or sunlight acts as the source of illumination. The light rays are reflected by a plane and concave mirror provided at the base.

Stage: It consists of a horizontal platform on which the object to be examined is mounted. It has a central aperture which allows the reflected light rays to fall on the object. A mechanical stage is fitted to the fixed stage so that the object can be moved from side to side or from front to back.

Sub-stage: This lies below the stage and it consists of a condenser and an iris diaphragm. The condenser consists of lenses which condenses and focuses the light rays from the mirror on to the object. The condenser can be lowered or raised by means of a knob at the side. The iris diaphragm can be used to control the amount of light reaching the object.

Body tube: At the upper end of the body tube, there is detachable eyepiece (X10). The lower end of it has a revolving nosepiece which carries three objective lenses of various magnifications as given below:

Objective lens	Magnification	Working distance	Numerical aperture
Low power	X10	5–6 mm	0.3
High power	X40	0.5–1.5 mm	0.6
Oil immersion	X100	0.15–0.20 mm	1.3

The oil immersion lens has the least working length and the highest magnification. It is so called because it has to be used with a drop of oil having the same refractive index as that of the glass slide so as to minimize the loss of light rays coming from the object. Cedar wood oil is commonly used as its refractive index is 1.515 which is the same as that of glass.

Focus adjustment knobs: Two such knobs are present at the side of the microscope. The bigger knob is used for coarse focusing and the smaller knob is used for fine focusing. Using these knobs the distance between the objective lens and the object can be adjusted so that the object lies at the focal length of the objective.

Magnification: Total magnifying power of the microscope = power of eyepiece × power of objective.

Focusing Procedures

Under Low Power

a. Place the slide to be focused on the stage and fit it into the mechanical stage.
b. Focus the light on the object by adjusting the plain mirror. Lower the objective (X10) and partially close the aperture.
c. The aperture of the objective lens is to be kept above the point that has to be focused on the slide.

d. The condenser should be lowered from the top position till the object is properly illuminated and focus is adjusted using the fine adjustment for a sharper focus.

For High Power Magnification

a. First focus under low power and select the required area.
b. Turn the high power objective lens into visualization position.
c. The iris diaphragm is to be fully opened and concave mirror is used to condense the light on the object.
d. Raise the condenser to high position.
e. Use the fine focusing knob to focus the object.

For Highest Magnification under Oil Immersion

a. First focus the slide under lower power and select a suitable area.
b. Place a drop of cedar wood oil over the selected site.
c. Turn the oil immersion lens into position.
d. Visualize under the plane mirror and open the iris diaphragm fully.
e. Raise the condenser to the highest position and by fine focusing knob focus the object.

PRECAUTIONS

1. Clean the eyepiece and objective lens gently with xylene before using the microscope.
2. After using the oil immersion lens, it should be cleaned with cotton soaked in xylol.
3. Do not lower the optical tube when you are looking through the eyepiece.
4. Support the base of the microscope and hold it uprightly while lifting it.

DENTAL IMPLICATIONS

The design and lens arrangement differs for the compound and surgical microscope, but as a student the observational and positional ergonomic skills are developed as they practice and work with the microscope.

Microscopic dentistry in practice provides very high levels of magnification and this helps in making precise diagnosis and provides effective dental care to the patient. As a dentist working with magnification, they are less likely to leave decay rather than managing patients without use of magnification. Dental operating microscope helps to identify, classify and successfully handle cracks in the dentin and enamel. The endodontic procedures are performed with dental operating microscope at a magnification ranging from X2.5 (access) to X20 (exploration or surgery), restorative dentistry surgery at magnification ranging from X2.5 to X19 and periodontal microsurgeries under X10 to X20 magnification. The student should note that the range in magnification vary depends on the type of microscope used and the components used.

OBJECTIVE STRUCTURED PRACTICAL EXAMINATION (OSPE) QUESTIONS

Focus the given slide under low power/high power/oil immersion lens under the provided microscope.

1. Picking the slide and appropriately placing it on the mechanical stage, adjusting the slide on the central aperture. (Yes/No)

2. Users the light source appropriately (plane/concave mirror). (Yes/No)

3. Identify the objective lens power appropriately. Low power lens (X10), high power lens (X40) or oil immersion lens (X100). (Yes/No)

4. Placement of the condenser accurately. Low power lens (X10), high power lens (X40) or oil immersion lens (X100) (Yes/No)

5. Using the fine focusing knob focuses the object. (Yes/No)

VIVA QUESTIONS

1. **Define numerical aperture, working distance and resolving power of the lens.**

Ans. The numerical aperture is a measure of the amount of light entering the objective lens. Working distance is roughly equal to the focal length and resolving power of lens gives the minimum separable distance between two points on the object which can be seen as two separate points.

$$\text{Minimum separable difference} = \frac{0.61 \times \text{wavelength of light}}{\text{Numerical aperture}}$$

2. **What will happen to image under focus if the aperture of oil immersion objective lens is more than a pinhole aperture?**

Ans. In case, the aperture of oil immersion lens is more than a pinhole spherical and chromatic aberration would distort the image.

3. **Which are the desired positions of condenser for seeing object in low power, high power and oil immersion?**

Ans. The desired position of the condenser is as follows:

Objective lens power	Condenser position
(i) Low power (X10)	(i) Lowest
(ii) High power (X40)	(ii) Higher [in between (i) and (iii)]
(iii) Oil immersion (X100)	(iii) Highest

4. **What is phase contrast microscopy?**

Ans. The phase contrast microscopy is an optical microscopy illumination technique, in which small phase shifts in the light passing through a transparent specimen

are converted into amplitude or contrast changes in the image. This microscope technique made it possible to study the cell cycle in live cells.

5. Name the variants of the electron microscopes.

Ans. The major variants of electron microscopes are scanning electron microscope (SEM) and transmission electron microscope (TEM).

6. Where will be the condenser position for low power and oil immersion lenses?

Ans. Low power lens permit the largest amount of light as the aperture of the lens is largest, hence the condenser position is placed low so that the brightness is low and it does not interfere with clarity of image.

While using the oil immersion lens, condenser should be raised right up to the stage, so that it intensify the illumination and the aperture of the iris—diaphragm is to be widely opened so as to allow the maximum light.

MULTIPLE CHOICE QUESTIONS

1. **Oil for visualization under oil immersion lens is:**
   A. Cedar wood oil
   B. Olive oil
   C. Sunflower oil
   D. Coconut oil

2. **Nobel Prize in Physics in 1986 was awarded for discovering scanning tunneling microscopy to:**
   A. Zaccharias Janssen
   B. Anton van Leeuwenhoek
   C. Heinrich Rohrer
   D. Gerd Binnig

3. **The maximum illumination on focused slide is obtained by:**
   A. Using the concave mirror with the condenser up and the iris-diaphragm open
   B. Using the convex mirror with the condenser up and the iris-diaphragm open
   C. Using the plain mirror with the condenser up and the iris-diaphragm open
   D. None of the above

4. **Optical tube's length is:**
   A. 25–26 mm
   B. 215–216 mm
   C. 125–126 mm
   D. 250–260 mm

5. **Objective lens power of oil immersion lens is:**
   A. X25
   B. X10
   C. X40
   D. X100

Answers:

| 1 A | 2 C, D | 3 A | 4 D | 5 D |

HISTORICAL ASPECT

Anton van Leeuwenhoek (1632–1723)

The father of microscopy, Anton van Leeuwenhoek of Holland, worked as an apprentice in a dry goods store where magnifying glasses were used to count the threads in cloth. Anton van Leeuwenhoek mastered new methods for grinding and polishing tiny lenses of great curvature which gave magnifications up to 270 diameters. These led to the discovery of his microscope. He made several biological discoveries, he was the first to see and describe bacteria, yeast plants, the teeming life in a drop of water and the circulation of blood corpuscles in capillaries.

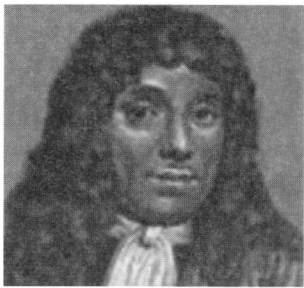

Anton van Leeuwenhoek

Robert Hooke

He was the English father of microscopy, reconfirmed Anton van Leeuwenhoek's discoveries of the existence of tiny living organisms in a drop of water. Hooke made a copy of Leeuwenhoek's light microscope and then improved upon his design.

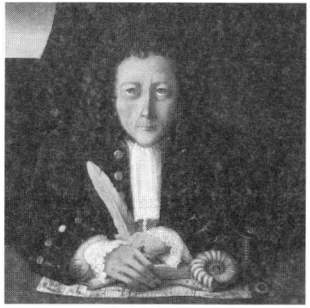

Robert Hooke

James Hillier

Physicist James Hillier is recognized for his contributions to the development of the electron microscope. Hillier's work on the electron microscope began in college. He and a fellow graduate student built a model in 1937 that magnified 7,000 times.

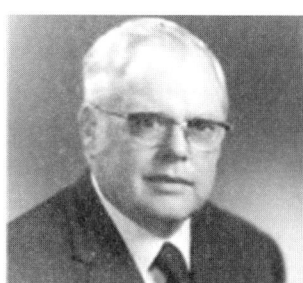

James Hillier

Gerd Binnig

He along with his colleague, Heinrich Rohrer, was awarded the Nobel Prize in Physics in 1986 for his work in scanning tunneling microscopy. Binnig and Rohrer developed the powerful microscopy technique that could form an image of individual atoms on a semiconductor surface or metal by scanning the tip of a needle over the surface at a height of only a few atomic diameters. They shared the Nobel Prize in Physics in 1986 with German scientist Ernst Ruska, designer of the first electron microscope.

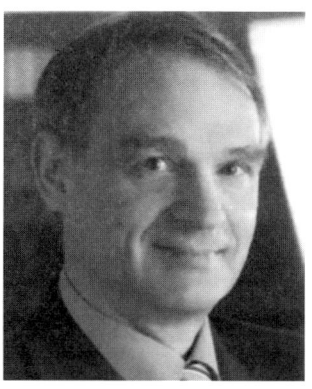

Gerd Binnig

RECENT UPDATES

The scanning tunneling microscope (STM) is being used in both industrial and fundamental research for obtaining atomic-scale images of metal surfaces. It provides a three-dimensional profile of the surface and helps for characterizing surface roughness, identifying surface defects, and evaluating the size and conformation of molecules and aggregates on the surface. The electrochemical scanning tunneling microscope was invented in 1988 by Kingo Itaya in Japan, and this helps to observe the structures of surfaces and electrochemical reactions in solid–liquid interfaces at atomic or molecular scales.

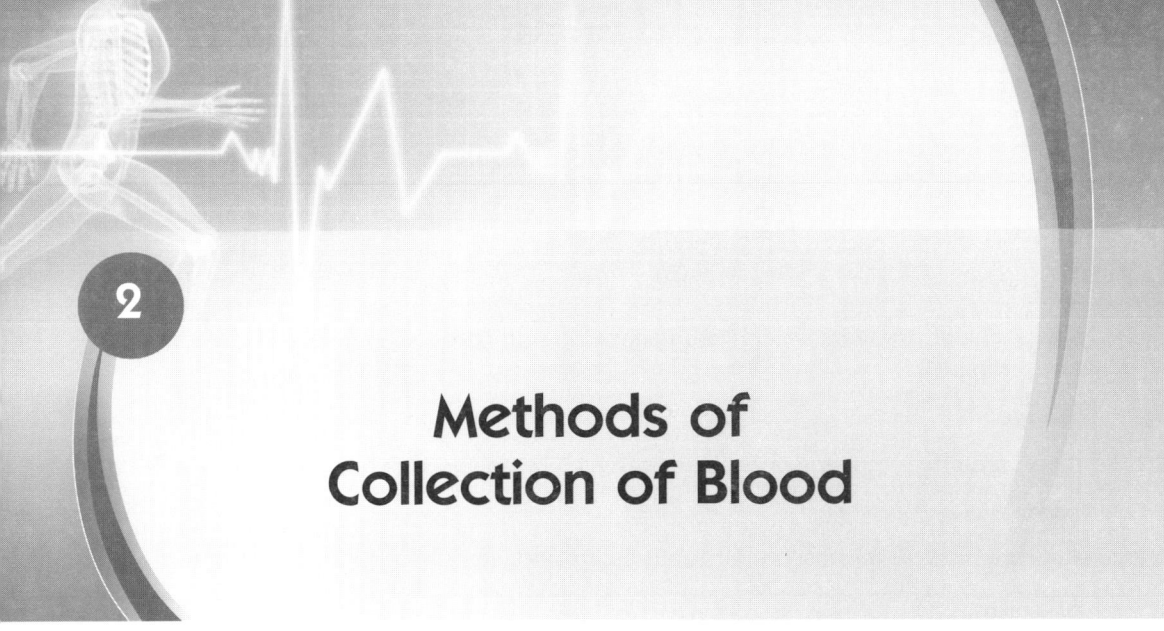

Methods of Collection of Blood

Learning Objectives
After the experiment the student should be able to:
1. Discuss the various methods of collecting a blood sample.
2. Describe the common anticoagulants used *in vitro* and *in vivo*.
3. Able to draw capillary and venous blood.

INTRODUCTION

Anticoagulants prevent blood coagulation and allow separation of the blood into liquid (plasma) and cellular components. The plasma contains coagulation factors. The common anticoagulants used are—3.8% trisodium citrate, potassium oxalate, EDTA (ethylenediaminetetraaceticacid), heparin, potassium ammonium oxalate and dicoumerol.

Trisodium Citrate

It prevents clotting of blood as it causes Ca^{++} to precipitate out as calcium citrate rendering Ca^{++} ions unavailable for clotting. It is the anticoagulant of choice for coagulation studies, and for estimation of erythrocyte sedimentation rate (ESR).

Potassium Oxalate

It reacts with calcium in the blood and forms an insoluble calcium complex thus making Ca^{++} ions unavailable for clotting. It is not commonly used as it causes shrinking of red blood cell (RBC).

Potassium Ammonium Oxalate

In the double oxalate mixture, potassium oxalate causes shrinking of RBC while ammonium oxalate causes swelling of RBC. This opposing effect of the two salts maintains the volume of the RBCs. Hence it is used as an anticoagulant for the determination of packed cell volume (PCV).

EDTA

It is a chelating agent which sequesters calcium, thereby making it unavailable for clotting.

Heparin

It is a naturally occurring anticoagulant which can be used both *in vivo* and *in vitro*. It facilitates the action of antithrombin III in binding and removing clotting factors IX, X, XI and XII. Hence they are not available for the formation of prothrombin activator and thrombin. In the absence of thrombin, fibrinogen cannot be converted to fibrin.

Dicoumarol

It is a vitamin K antagonist. Vitamin K is necessary for the formation of clotting factors II, VII, IX and X in the liver. Dicoumarol as a vitamin K antagonist prevents the formation of these factors and prevents clotting. It can be used only *in vivo*.

METHODS OF COLLECTION OF BLOOD SAMPLE

Materials: Disposable sterile, lancet, 5 mL syringe, 20 gauze needle, cotton and spirit.

Collection of Capillary Blood Sample

This site for collecting capillary blood is from fingertip and earlobe in an adult and from the ball of the heel in infants.

Finger Prick Method
• Clean the ring or middle finger with a spirit swab.
• Prick the fingertip using aseptic precaution using a sterile lancet.
• The prick should be deep enough to ensure a free flow of blood.
• Do not squeeze the finger to obtain blood.
• The first drop of blood is to be wiped with sterile cotton.
• The subsequent drop is utilized to conduct various estimation [for example, white blood cell (WBC) count, red blood cell (RBC) count, bleeding time and clotting time, etc].

Pricking the Earlobe

Gently rub the earlobe to make it warm, make a single firm prick to a depth of 2–3 mm with a sterile needle of 22/23 gauze. Wipe away the first few drops and collect the sample as the blood starts flowing freely.

Pricking the Heel

This method is used to obtain sample of blood in infants. Warm the heel by gentle rub and then give a deep prick on the lateral or medical parts of the plantar surface of the heel.

Collection of Venous Blood

Venous blood for hematological examinations can be obtained from the antecubital vein.

- The subject is asked to sit comfortably with his/her arm resting on the table.
- Identify a vein in the antecubital fossa.
- Apply a tourniquet around the upper arm and ask the subject to close his/her fist firmly in order to make the vein prominent.
- Clean the skin over the selected area with spirit and allow it to dry.
- Take a sterile dry 5 mL syringe with a 21 or 22 gauze needle and introduce the tip of the needle under the skin near the vein and puncture the vein from the side; taking care to avoid a counter puncture.

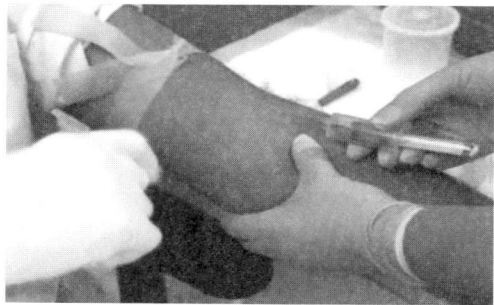

Fig. 2.1 Collection of venous blood sample

- When blood flows into the syringe, release the tourniquet and draw the required amount of blood.
- The needle should be withdrawn gently. Using a sterile cotton swab apply pressure for 2–3 minutes at the site of puncture to prevent blood loss.
- Remove the needle from the syringe and deliver the blood into a sterile container containing anticoagulant.
- Mix the blood with the anticoagulant by shaking the closed bottle gently over the table.
- Rinse the needle and syringe with water and arrange for disposal.

DENTAL IMPLICATION

The knowledge of anticoagulants and collection of blood trains the students to appropriately collect blood sample for investigations. Understanding the clotting mechanism and role of anticoagulant, the dental surgeons are alert while managing patients with coagulopathies. When performing the invasive procedure, the dental surgeon needs to follow the standard recommended protocol for minimizing tissue trauma and consideration of hemostatic systems for preventing extensive bleeding during surgical procedures; especially for patients with coagulopathies. The importance of having physician consultation and drug dose modification in patients on anticoagulation therapy is very much required while conducting dental procedures or surgery.

OBJECTIVE STRUCTURED PRACTICAL EXAMINATION (OSPE) QUESTIONS

Collection of Venous Blood

The subject is sitting comfortably with his/her arm resting on the table.

1. Identify a vein in the antecubital fossa. (Yes/No)

2. Apply a tourniquet around the upper arm and ask the subject to (Yes/No) close his/her fist firmly in order to make the vein prominent.

3. Clean the skin over the selected area with spirit. Taking a sterile dry (Yes/No) 5 mL syringe with a 21/22 gauze needle and introducing the tip of the needle under the skin near the vein and puncturing the vein from the side avoiding a counter puncture.

4. When blood flows into the syringe releasing the tourniquet and (Yes/No) drawing the required amount of blood.

5. The needle gently withdrawn. Applying a sterile cotton swab and (Yes/No) asking the subject to apply pressure for 2–3 minutes at the site of puncture to prevent blood loss.

6. Removing the needle from the syringe and delivering the blood (Yes/No) into a sterile container containing anticoagulant.

7. Mixing the blood with the anticoagulant by shaking the closed bottle (Yes/No) gently over the table.

8. Rinsing the needle and syringe with water and disposing the needle (Yes/No) in the disposal container.

VIVA QUESTIONS

1. How should the needle, syringe and blood sample be disposed?

Ans. The needle and syringe must be disposed of in approved sharps disposal containers. Other contaminated waste must be discarded in an appropriate biohazard bag.

2. Which toxic symptoms may occur because of sodium oxalate ingestion?

Ans. It can cause burning pain in the mouth, throat and stomach, bloody vomiting, headache, muscle cramps, convulsions, hypotension, heart failure, shock, coma and possible death. Mean lethal dose by ingestion of oxalates is 10–15 grams [per material safety data sheet (MSDS)].

3. What is the role of EDTA in chelation therapy?

Ans. EDTA is used to bind metal ions in the practice of chelation therapy, e.g. for treating mercury and lead poisoning. It is also used to remove excess iron from the body.

4. Which of the market products have EDTA as a component?

Ans. Shampoos, cleaners and other personal care products have EDTA salts as component and are used as a sequestering agent to improve their stability in air.

5. When was sodium citrate used as anticoagulant in blood transfusion?

Ans. Belgian doctor Albert Hustin and Argentine physician Luis Agote successfully used sodium citrate as anticoagulant in blood transfusions in 1914.

6. What is the role of sodium citrate in coagulation?

Ans. The citrate ion chelates calcium ions in the blood by forming calcium citrate complexes, disrupting the blood clotting mechanism.

7. Where from is heparin produced in the human body?

Ans. Yes, heparin is a naturally occurring anticoagulant produced by basophils and mast cells.

8. Explain the mechanism of anticoagulant effect of heparin.

Ans. It facilitates the action of antithrombin III, by binding and removing clotting factors IX, X, XI and XII. Hence these clotting factors are not available for the formation of prothrombin activator and thrombin. In the absence of thrombin, fibrinogen cannot be converted to fibrin.

MULTIPLE CHOICE QUESTIONS

1. **The personal protective equipment that should be worn in hematology laboratory is:**
   - **A.** Laboratory coat
   - **B.** Gloves
   - **C.** Mask
   - **D.** All of the above

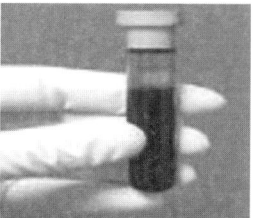

Photo (Q 2)

2. **The photo in the picture contains:**
   - **A.** Whole blood
   - **B.** Serum
   - **C.** Plasma
   - **D.** Saliva

3. **Identify the object in the photo:**
   - **A.** Disposable syringe
   - **B.** Plastic bottle
   - **C.** Stirrer
   - **D.** Piston

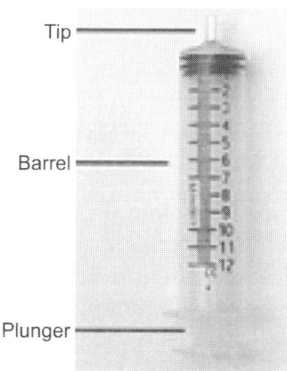

Tip

Barrel

Plunger

Photo (Q 3)

4. **Identify the object in the photo:**
   A. Needle used along with syringe for drawing blood. They are of various sizes (needle of 21 or 22 gauze is preferably used)
   B. Lancet
   C. Forceps
   D. Scalpel

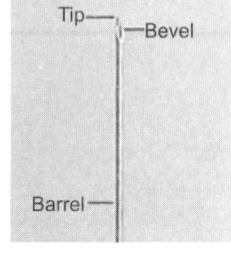

Photo (Q 4)

5. **EDTA was first described and prepared from the compound ethylenediamine and chloroacetic acid by:**
   A. Ferdinand Munz
   B. Albert Hustin
   C. Robert Cook
   D. Alferd Criks

Answers:

1 D	2 A	3 A	4 A	5 A

HISTORICAL ASPECT

The major breakthrough in discovery of Vacutainer tube, Auto Analyzer and electrophoresis occurred between the years of 1948 to 1960. The Vacutainer tube is designed to fill predetermined volume of blood by vacuum. Joseph J Kleiner (1897–1974) developed the first interchangeable syringe. Kleiner in 1943 planned to design multifit syringe and in 1952, Becton Dickinson and Company introduced multifit syringes engineered precisely with totally interchangeable parts. The blood collection tubes are drawn in a specific recommended order to avoid cross-contamination of additives between the tubes; for example, blood culture bottle or tube (yellow/yellow-black top), EDTA (lavender top), coagulation tube (light blue top), lithium heparin anticoagulant and a gel separator (light green top), oxalate/fluoride (light gray top), acid citrate dextrose (pale yellow top), etc.

RECENT UPDATES

In routine dental practice, fingerprick or fingerstick are commonly conducted on capillary blood for estimation of blood sugar, hemoglobin level, complete blood count, prothrombin time, etc. Fingersticks are sometimes carried out in children and the elderly, when small amount of blood (less than 500 µg) is required for a test. The fingerstick testing is also used to test for mononucleosis.

The venous blood is sucked up in a capillary tube on principle of surface tension or even by indirect suction.

The following procedures are to be meticulously followed for fingerstick test:

1. The patient is positioned in sitting or lying down position and his arm is hyperextend.
2. Fingersticks are carried out commonly on the 3rd (middle) and 4th (ring) fingers of the non-dominant hand using a sterile lancet.
3. The first drop of blood is wiped out as it contains excess tissue fluid.
4. After a drop of blood freely oozes out at fingertips, collect the blood into the collection device.
5. After capping and rotating, the collection device is inverted to mix the blood.
6. The patient should be asked to hold a gauze pad over the puncture site for a couple of minutes to stop the bleeding.
7. Ensure labelling tubes appropriately for sending it to the lab.
8. If sticks are used for glucose estimation, place the stick in the calibrated glucometer and note the value.

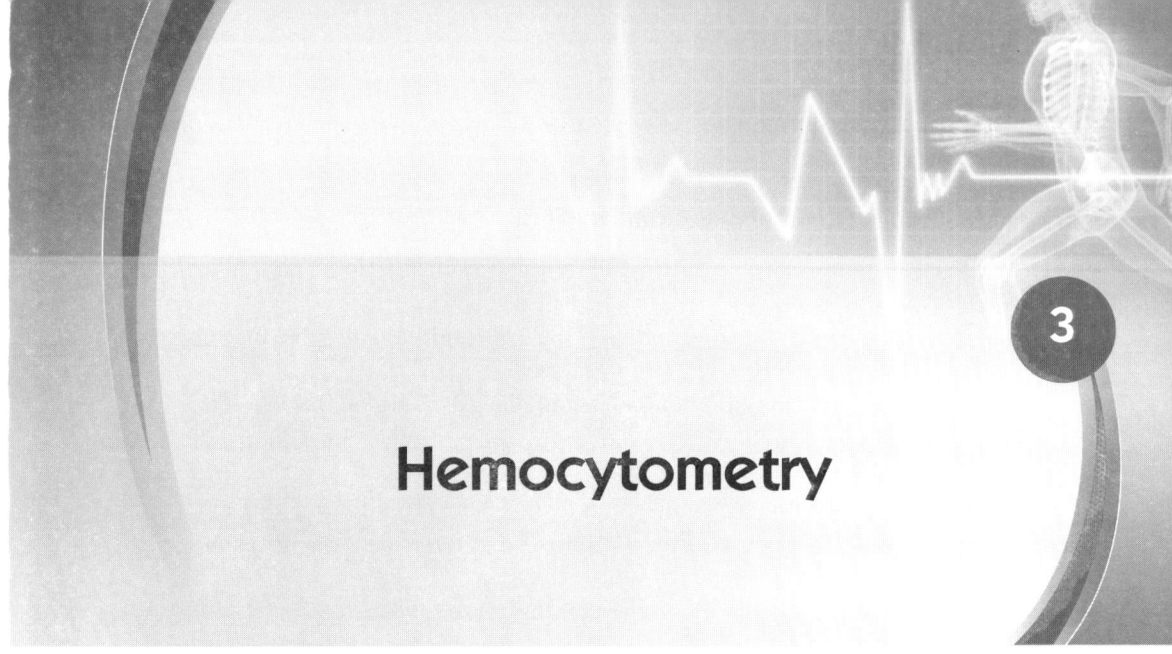

Hemocytometry

MATERIALS AND CHEMICALS

Lancet for making a sterile finger prick, hemacytometer with cover slip (improved Neubauer counting chamber), WBC and RBC pipettes, WBC and RBC diluting fluids and microscope.

RBC Pipette

It consists of a stem which widens into a bulb carrying a red bead. The stem is graduated and has two markings: (1) 0.5 and (2) 1.0 marks. Stem is followed by bulb which carries the red bead, and the bulb narrows above and has 101 as mark on it. This end is connected to a rubber tube which ends as mouthpiece. The red bead presence in the bulb along with markings helps in identifying the RBC pipette. The function of the red bead is to facilitate mixing in the bulb.

WBC Pipette

It is similar to the RBC pipette but has a smaller bulb capacity and a white bead inside. The graduations are 0.5 and 1 on the stem and 11 above the bulb. The rubber tubing from the bulb ends in a white mouthpiece.

Hemocytometer

It consists of a thick glass slide divided into two mirror-coated central platforms by an H-shaped groove. The central platform is slightly lower than the side platforms. The cover slip is placed on the side platforms and covers the central platform. The distance between the cover slip and the central platform is 1/10 mm.

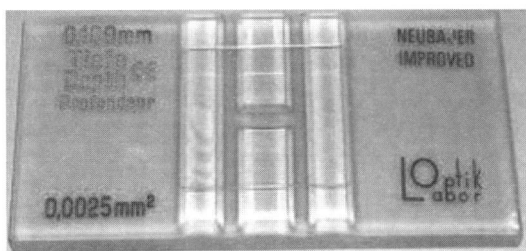

Fig. 3.1 Neubauer chamber

The central platform has lines engraved on both sides to form squares of different dimensions which are used for different cell counts. The total ruled area consists of a square having a dimension of 3 × 3 mm which is divided into nine squares each having an area of 1 sq mm (1 × 1 mm). The nine squares comprises four corner squares which are used for the WBC count and the central square for the RBC count. Each WBC square is further divided into 16 squares of 1/16 sq mm.

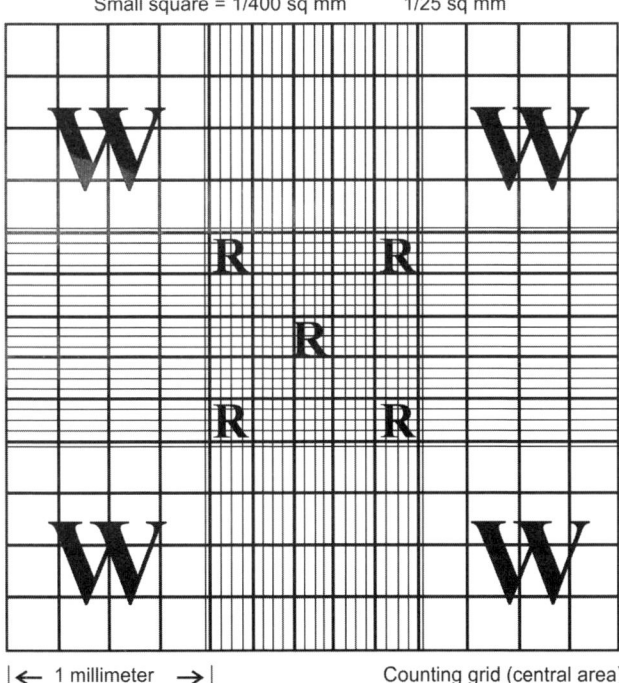

Fig. 3.2 Counting grid of improved Neubauer ruling. RBCs are counted in five groups of 25 medium-sized squares etched in central large square. WBCs are counted in four large corner square

The central large RBC square is divided into 25 medium-sized squares by triple lines. Each medium-sized square has an area of $1/5 \times 1/5$ mm = $1/25$ sq mm. The central medium-sized square and four corner medium-sized squares are used for the RBC count. The area of the 5 medium-sized square is $1/25 \times 5 = 1/5$ sq mm. As the depth under the cover slip is $1/10$ mm, the volume of five of the medium-sized squares is $1/5 \times 1/10 = 1/50$ cu mm.

The medium sized squares are further divided into 16 small squares, i.e. $25 \times 16 = 400$ small squares. The side of the smallest RBC square is $1/20$ mm. The area of the smallest RBC square is $1/20 \times 1/20 = 1/400$ sq mm. As the depth under the cover slip is $1/10$ mm, the volume of the smallest RBC square is $1/400 \times 1/10 = 1/4,000$ cu mm. RBCs are counted in 80 small squares. Therefore, the volume of 80 small size RBC squares is $1/4,000 \times 80 = 1/50$ cu mm.

METHOD

Study the Neubauer's chamber and identify the squares for the RBC and WBC counts under the compound microscope. Study the squares under low power and then under high power. Identify the WBC and RBC pipette. Practice drawing the fluid in the pipette. Practice charging the Neubauer's chamber.

Dilution for RBC Count

- Take a clean and dry pipette.
- Pour the RBC diluting fluid (hayem's fluid) in a watch glass.
- Clean the middle or the index finger with spirit. Give a finger prick using lancet, and then suck blood up to the 0.5 mark. No air bubbles should accumulate during the process.
- Wipe the tip of the pipette using sterile gauze, and then suck Hayem's fluid up to the 101 mark.
- Keep the pipette initially at an acute angle while sucking in the Hayem's fluid and then gradually make it vertical as the fluid reaches the 101 mark.
- Place the pipette in a horizontal position and firmly hold the index finger of one hand over the opening in the tip of the pipette, close the rubber end of the pipette by tying a gentle knot using the other hand. Ensure that the pipette is in a horizontal position.
- Mix the contents of the bulb between the palms of the two hands gently.
- As 0.5 parts of blood are diluted in 100 parts of Hayem's fluid, the dilution achieved is of $1:200$.
- Discard the fluid in the stem as it contains only diluting fluid.

Dilution for WBC Count

1. Draw the blood up to 0.5 mark in the WBC pipette.
2. Wipe the outside of the capillary pipette to remove excess blood that would interfere with the dilution factor.

3. Holding the pipette almost vertical place into the fluid. Draw the diluting fluid into the pipette slowly until the mixture reaches the 11 mark while gently rotating the pipette to ensure a proper amount of mixing.

4. Place the pipette in a horizontal position and firmly hold the index finger of one hand over the opening in the tip of the pipette, close the rubber end of the pipette by tying a gentle knot using the other hand. Ensure that the pipette is in a horizontal position.

5. Mix the sample for at least 3 minutes to facilitate hemolysis of RBCs.

6. This can be accomplished by drawing the blood up to 1.0 mark and the diluting fluid to the 11 mark. The dilution will then be $1:10$ and the dilution factor in the calculation will be 10.

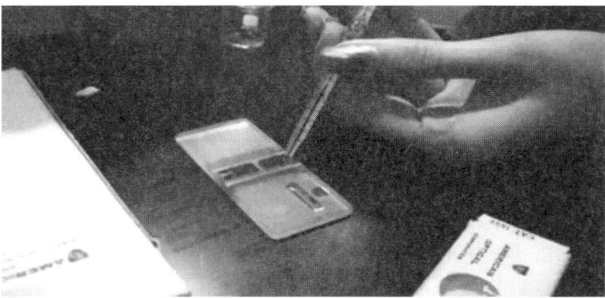

Fig. 3.3 Charging of Neubauer's chamber

Charging the Improved Neubauer's Chamber

1. Clean the hemacytometer and its cover slip with an alcohol pad and wait for 2 minutes to make it dry.

2. Discard first three to four drops of the mixture on a piece of gauze so as to expel the diluent from the stem.

3. The tip of the pipette is to be placed on the central platform at an angle of 45° near the edge of the cover slip and carefully allow a small amount of fluid to flow under the cover slip.

4. Ensure that no air bubbles are present and there is no overflow of fluid into the grooves.

5. After charging allow the cells to settle and then focus the cells and the squares under the microscope.

DENTAL IMPLICATION

In dental practice and prior to dental surgery or dental procedures RBC, WBC and differential leukocyte count is required to diagnose anemia or ensure the immunity status. These investigations can be done using Neubauer's chamber in dental clinic or dental indoor unit. Hence the skills of estimation of cell count using hemocytometer should be mastered.

OBJECTIVE STRUCTURED PRACTICAL EXAMINATION (OSPE) QUESTIONS

Charge the Neubauer chamber with the given diluted fluid in the pipette

1. The tip of the pipette is placed on the central platform at an angle   (Yes/No)
   of 45° near the edge of the cover slip and carefully allows a small
   amount of fluid to flow under the cover slip.
2. Ensures that no air bubbles are present and there is no overflow   (Yes/No)
   of fluid into the grooves.

Additional OSPE Questions for Practice

• Focus an RBC counting square in the Neubauer chamber under 40X
• Dilute the given sample of blood for total WBC count
• Dilute the given sample of blood for RBC count
• Focus a WBC counting square under high power

VIVA QUESTIONS

1. **Who invented the hemocytometer?**

Ans. Louis-Charles Malassez invented the hemocytometer.

2. **Describe the gridded area of hemocytometer.**

Ans. Hemocytometer has nine 1×1 mm (1 mm^2) squares in the girdded area which
are subdivided in three dimensions: 0.25×0.20 mm (0.05 mm^2), 0.25×0.25 mm
(0.0625 mm^2), and 0.20×0.20 mm (0.04 mm^2) and the central square is subdivided
into 0.05×0.05 mm (0.0025 mm^2) squares.

3. **Name the two common applications of hemocytometer.**

Ans. The two common applications of hemocytometer include its use for blood count
and sperm count.

4. **How will you adjust the blood level if it is drawn above the mark 0.5 in the
   RBC or WBC pipette?**

Ans. The blood level if drawn above the mark 0.5 can be adjusted to the correct level
by tapping the tip of the pipette against the fingernail or by touch the tip of the
pipette with a non-absorbent material.

5. **Why do we discard the first two drops from the RBC or WBC pipette before
   charging the Neubauer chamber?**

Ans. The first two drops from the RBC or WBC pipette are discarded before charging
the Neubauer chamber as they contain only the diluting fluid.

6. **What are the features of RBC diluting pipette?**

Ans. The features of RBC diluting pipette are:
   • The markings on the pipette include 0.5, 1 and 101.
   • The luminal diameter of the stem of RBC pipette is smaller when compared to
     that of WBC pipette.

- The bulb contains a red bead.
- The volume of the bulb of the RBC pipette is larger than that of the WBC pipette.

7. **How does the old Neubauer chamber differ from the improved Neubauer chamber?**

Ans. The central (1 mm^2) large square in the old Neubauer chamber contains 16 medium-sized squares separated by triple lines in comparison to the 25 medium-sized squares which are separated by double or triple lines in the improved Neubauer chamber.

8. **Why should the tip of the pipette be wiped off before sucking the diluting fluid?**

Ans. The tip of the pipette should be wiped off before sucking the diluting fluid to prevent the entry of the extra drop blood from entering into the pipette which may give rise to false high cell counts and to avoid contamination of the diluting fluid.

MULTIPLE CHOICE QUESTIONS

1. **The function of the bead in the RBC and WBC pipette includes all of the following except**
   - **A.** To facilitate mixing of the contents in the bulb
   - **B.** Helps to distinguish the RBC and WBC pipette
   - **C.** Prevents clotting of blood
   - **D.** Indicates the dryness of the pipette

2. **Which among the following is incorrect regarding the WBC pipette?**
   - **A.** The markings on the pipette include 0.5, 1 and 11
   - **B.** The luminal diameter of the stem of WBC pipette is smaller when compared to that of RBC pipette.
   - **C.** The bulb contains a white bead
   - **D.** The volume of the bulb of the WBC pipette is smaller than that of the RBC pipette.

3. **The depth under the coverslip in the improved Neubauer chamber is**
   - **A.** 0.1 mm
   - **B.** 0.01 mm
   - **C.** 0.001 mm
   - **D.** 0.0001 mm

4. **The following statements are true, except**
   - **A.** The tip of the pipette should be dipped into the blood drop to avoid the entry of air bubbles.
   - **B.** Blood if drawn above the mark 0.5, can be adjusted to the correct level using cotton swabs.
   - **C.** Tip of the pipette should be wiped before dipping it into the diluting fluid.
   - **D.** Dilution of blood with the respective diluting fluid must be done quickly to avoid clotting of blood.

5. **Which among the following is incorrect regarding charging of the Neubauer chamber?**

   A. The chamber must be completely covered by the diluting fluid.

   B. If the chamber is overcharged, it must be washed, dried and recharged again.

   C. The first two drops of fluid in the pipette must be discarded before charging the Neubauer chamber.

   D. The cells must be counted immediately after charging the Neubauer chamber.

Answers:				
1 C	2 B	3 A	4 B	5 C

HISTORICAL ASPECT

Louis-Charles Malassez (1842–1909)

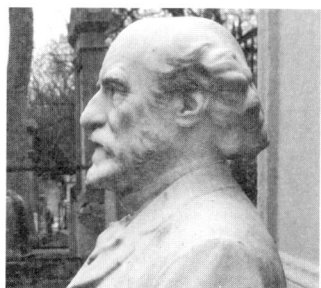

Louis-Charles Malassez, born on September 21 1842, was a French Anatomist.

Malassez is known for his studies of microscopic anatomy, histology of blood cells as well as for inventing the hemacytometer. In dentistry, he studied some ligament cells which are now named after him, called the epithelial cell rests of Malassez (ERM). A genus of fungi *Malassezia* is also named after him and includes species that can cause skin irritation.

Louis-Charles Malassez

RECENT UPDATES

Though utility of the manual hemocytometers cannot be sidelined as it interprets results by human eye observation; but with increased work load in labs the automated cell counters are now being used for sampling the blood and describing cell populations using electrical and optical techniques for counts of RBCs, WBCs and platelets. The advanced cell counters today also report Cell Population Data within the Leukocyte morphological information and clue for suspecting diseases on the basis of observed cell abnormalities. Reticulocyte counts today are assessed with modern analysers, using supravital dye such as new methylene blue and these analysers also have has a modular slide maker for producing a blood film of consistent quality and stain the film.

Procedures of Hematology

- Enumeration of red blood cells count
- Enumeration of white blood cells count
- Differential leukocyte count
- Determination of hemoglobin
- Determination of blood groups (A, B, O and Rh system)
- Determination of bleeding time and clotting time
- Clinical examination of radial pulse
- Recording of systemic arterial blood pressure

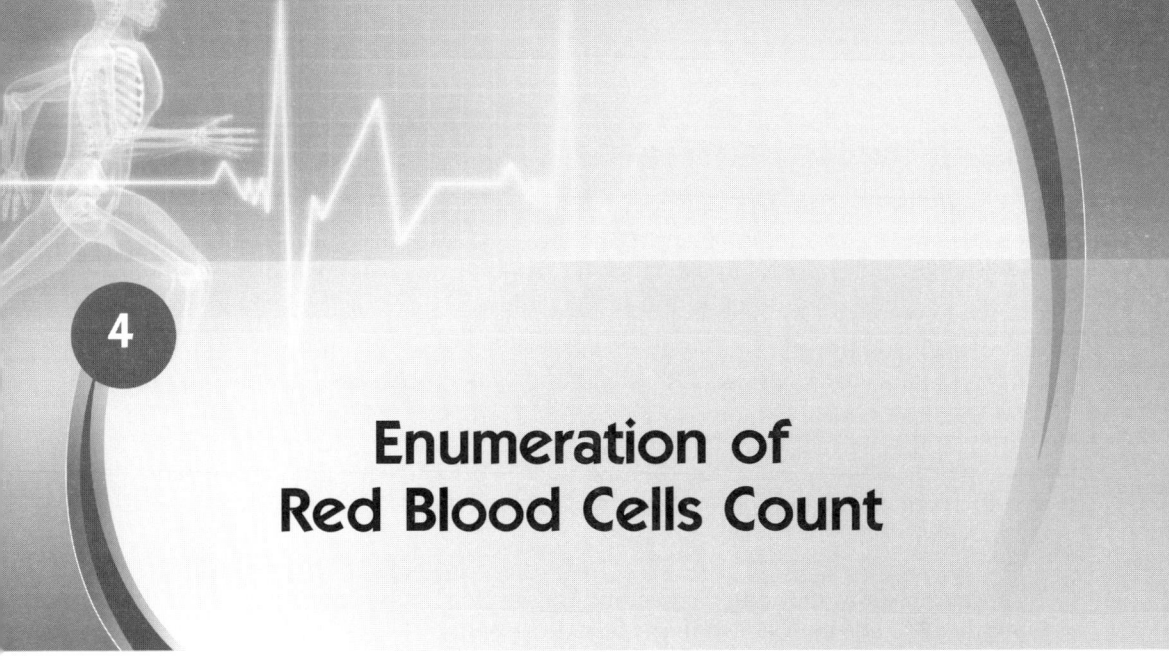

Enumeration of Red Blood Cells Count

Learning Objectives

After completion of practicals, the student should be able to:
1. Identify the red blood cell pipette and draw the blood and diluent.
2. Charge the Neubauer's chamber and carry red blood cell count.
3. Discuss the normal range of red blood cell and explain the causes of anemia.

INTRODUCTION

Red blood cells (RBCs) are the most common type of cells in the blood and are extremely important because they carry oxygen from the lungs to the body tissues. The RBC count ranges from 4.2 to 5 million per microliter of blood for women and 4.6–6.0 million for men. A normal RBC count for children is typically between 3.8 million and 5.5 million RBCs per volume. A decrease in RBC count is seen in anemia, acute or chronic blood loss, malnutrition, chronic inflammation, or a number of nutritional deficiencies including iron, copper, vitamin B_{12}, or vitamin B_6. It is biconcave in shape having a diameter of 7.8 micron and mean corpuscular volume of 90–95 cubic microns.

DENTAL PERSPECTIVE

Dental patients presenting with symptoms and signs (systemic as well as oral sign) of anemia should be recommended for a complete blood count (CBC). If hemoglobin levels are lowered significantly in patient, they should be referred to physician for a more thorough medical history, laboratory diagnosis and treatment. None of the elective oral surgical or periodontal procedures should be performed on patients with marked anemia because of the potential danger of increased bleeding and impaired wound healing. The decrease in hemoglobin levels below 10 g/dL leads to the low oxygen tension affecting the rheological interactions between the cellular components of blood, mainly platelets and endothelium and thereby decreasing their ability to clot effectively. The dental surgeon should not administer general anesthesia if the hemoglobin is at least 10 g/dL.

Aims: Enumeration of the number of erythrocytes in 1 cu mm of blood.

Materials and chemicals: Neubauer's chamber with cover slip, red cell pipette, microscope and diluting fluid [the diluting fluid is the Hayem's fluid and it contains mercuric chloride (0.5 gm); sodium chloride (1 gm); sodium sulphate (5 gm) dissolved in distill water of 200 mL].

Procedures

1. Take a clean and dry pipette.
2. Pour the RBC diluting fluid (Hayem's fluid) in a watch glass.
3. Clean the middle or the index finger with spirit. Give a finger prick using lancet, and then suck blood up to the 0.5 mark. No air bubbles should accumulate during the process.
4. Wipe the tip of the pipette using sterile gauze, and then suck Hayem's fluid up to the 101 mark.
5. Keep the pipette initially at an acute angle while sucking in the Hayem's fluid and then gradually make it vertical as the fluid reaches the 101 mark.
6. Place the pipette in a horizontal position and firmly hold the index finger of one hand over the opening in the tip of the pipette, close the rubber end of the pipette by tying a gentle knot using the other hand. Ensure that the pipette is in a horizontal position.
7. Mix the contents of the bulb between the palms of the two hands gently. Discard the first few drops of pure diluting fluid present in the stem.

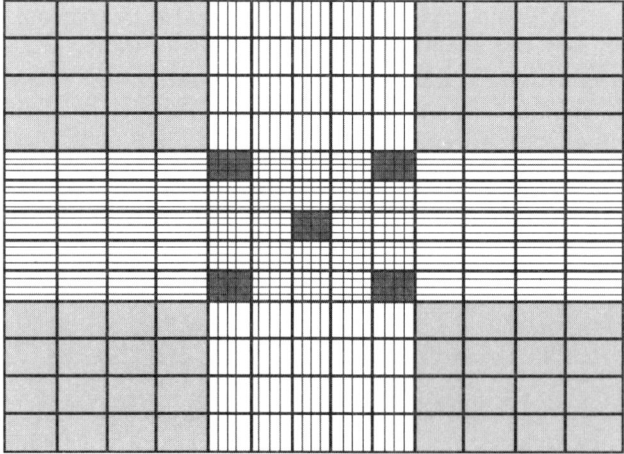

Fig. 4.1 Showing ▭ Areas of the grid where WBCs are counted
▨ Areas of the grid where RBCs are counted

8. Charge the Neubauer's chamber as instructed in practical of hemocytometry.

9. Allow time for cells to settle down and then start counting cell. Focus the chamber under low power and check for uniform distribution of cells. Focus the RBC square and identify the four corner squares and the center square under the high power objective.

10. **Counting:** Count the total number of RBCs in the four corner squares and in the central square (total of 5 medium-sized squares or $16 \times 5 = 80$ small squares).

Calculation

- Area of 5 medium-sized RBC squares = $1/25 \times 5 = 1/5$ sq mm.
- Depth under the cover slip = $1/10$ mm.
- Volume of 5 medium-sized squares = $1/5 \times 1/10 = 1/50$ cu mm.
- Number of cells in $1/50$ cu.mm volume of diluted blood = nRBCs. Therefore, 1 cu mm of diluted blood contains = $n \times 50/1$ RBCs.
- The dilution factor is $1:200$ (0.5 parts of blood in 100 parts of Hayem's fluid). Therefore, 1 cu mm of undiluted blood contains = $n \times 50/1 \times 200/1 = n \times 10,000$ RBCs.

Results: Record your observations and results.

DENTAL IMPLICATION

Patient reporting for dental problems may have anemia. This result from blood loss, destruction or reduced production of RBCs, fluid overload, vitamin and nutrient deficiencies, genetic disorders in hemoglobinopathies, etc. Hence treating patient for anemia with consultation of physician is advisable before any major oral procedures or surgery.

OBJECTIVE STRUCTURED PRACTICAL EXAMINATION (OSPE) QUESTIONS

Dilute the given sample of blood for RBC count

1. Sucks blood up to the 0.5 mark; ensure no air bubbles accumulate during the process. (Yes/No)

2. Wipes the tip of the pipette using sterile gauze, and then suck Hayem's fluid up to the 101 mark. (Yes/No)

3. Keeps the pipette initially at an acute angle while sucking in the Hayem's fluid and then gradually makes it vertical as the fluid reaches the 101 mark. (Yes/No)

4. Places the pipette in a horizontal position and firmly hold the index finger of one hand over the opening in the tip of the pipette, closes the rubber end of the pipette by tying a gentle knot using the other hand. Ensures that pipette is kept in horizontal position. (Yes/No)

5. Mixes the contents of the bulb between the palms of the two hands gently. Discards the first few drops of the diluting fluid of the stem of the pipette. (Yes/No)

Non-skilled OSPE I

1. **Enlist the elements and source required for red blood cell production.**

Ans. The elements and dietary sources for increasing red blood cell production are.
- Iron: Lentils and legumes
- Folic acid: Lentils, cereals fortified with folic acid and dark green leafy vegetables
- Copper: Shellfish, poultry, liver, beans, cherries, whole grains, nuts and chocolate
- Vitamin B_{12}: Meat, eggs and fortified cereals.
- Vitamin B_6: Meat, fish, whole grains, vegetables and legumes.
- Vitamin A: Grapefruit, watermelon, plums, mangoes and apricots.

Non-skilled OSPE II

1. **Enlist any three measures for increasing red blood cells.**

Ans. The three measures for increasing red blood cells are:
1. Exercise
2. Blood transfusions
3. Erythropoietin hormone therapy stimulates the bone marrow to increase red blood cells production especially useful in patients who are in kidney failure or receiving chemotherapy treatment.

VIVA QUESTIONS

1. **What is the average life span of the red blood cells? Where are they destroyed?**

Ans. The average life span of red blood cells live is around 120 days. The spleen is the main organ where old RBCs are destroyed.

2. **What are erythrocytes also known as? What are the functions of erythrocyte?**

Ans. Erythrocytes are also known as red blood cells or red blood corpuscles (RBCs). Erythrocytes are responsible for oxygen transport from the lungs to the tissues.

3. **What is anemia? What are the four main types of anemia?**

Ans. Anemia is low concentration of hemoglobin in the blood.

The four main types of anemia are:
1. Nutrient deficiency anemia,
2. Anemia caused by blood loss,
3. Hemolytic anemia and
4. Aplastic anemia.

1. **Nutrient deficiency anemia** is caused due to deficiency of fundamental nutrients for the production or functioning of the RBC in the diet and leads to deficiencies of iron (iron deficiency anemia), vitamin B_{12} and folic acid.

2. **Anemia caused by blood loss** occurs in hemorrhagic conditions, peptic ulcerations and hookworm diseases.

3. **Hemolytic anemia** is caused by excessive destruction of RBCs, for example, in diseases, defects of RBC membrane production (as in hereditary sperocytosis), defects in hemoglobin production (as in thalassemia and sickle-cell anemia), G6PD deficiency, hypersplenism, lead poisoning, etc.

4. **Aplastic anemia** occurs from deficiencies of the hematopoiesis and it happens when the bone marrow is injured by cancers from other tissues (metastasis), by autoimmune diseases and by intoxication from drugs (like sulfa and anticonvulsants) or by chemical substances (like benzene, insecticides, paints, herbicides and solvents in general). Some genetic diseases also affect the bone marrow causing aplastic anemia.

4. **What are the symptoms observed in patient of anemia?**

Ans. The symptoms observed in patients of anemia are fatigue, shortness of breath, palpitation, angina, intermittent claudication of legs, malaise, headache, etc.

MULTIPLE CHOICE QUESTIONS

1. **The average life span of an RBC is:**

   A. 50 days   **B.** 100 days

   C. 112 days   **D.** 120 days

2. **Which of these are the functions of RBC?**

   A. Helps in identifying blood groups

   B. Helps transport of gases

   C. Helps in maintaining acid base balance in the body

   D. All of the above

3. **At birth, RBCs are:**

   A. Larger in size

   B. More number of juvenile RBCs is observed

   C. RBC count is high

   D. All of the above

4. **Colony stimulating factor increases production of all except:**

   A. Neutrophils

   B. Lymphocytes

   C. Basophils

   D. Macrophages

5. **During development of RBC hemoglobin appears in the:**
   A. Intermediate normoblast stage
   B. Early normoblast stage
   C. Initial stage of late normoblast stage
   D. Final stage of late normoblast stage

6. **Most potent stimulus for production of RBCs is:**
   A. Blood loss   B. Bone marrow hypoxia
   C. Decrease in arterial pO_2 D. Bacterial infections

7. **Hypoxia of kidney causes immediate release of:**
   A. Erythropoietinogen   B. Renal erythropoietic factor
   C. Renin   D. Erythropoietin

8. **Hemaglobinuria in the morning is suggestive of**
   A. Paroxysmal nocturnal hemoglobinuria
   B. Nephritis
   C. Iron deficiency anemia
   D. Sickle cell anemia

9. **Intrinsic factor is secreted by:**
   A. Kidney   B. Chief cells of stomach
   C. Parietal cells of stomach D. Beta cells of pancreas

10. **Extrinsic factor required for maturation of RBCs is:**
    A. Vitamin B_{12} B. Folic acid
    C. Calcium   D. A and B both

Answers:

1 D	2 D	3 D	4 D	5 A	6 C	7 D	8 A
9 C	10 D						

CLINICAL CASE SCENARIO

1. **Which precautions will you take as a dentist while treating patient with polycythemia vera?**

Ans. As a dentist, you should have consultation with hematologist in planning and performing the dental treatment of your patient because of risk of blood clotting cascade attenuation while conducting dental procedure or surgery.

2. **What are the oral signs seen in patient of anemia due to vitamin B$_{12}$ and folate deficiency?**

Ans. The oral signs seen in patient of anemia due to vitamin B$_{12}$ and folate deficiency are angular stomatitis, glossitis and candidal infections.

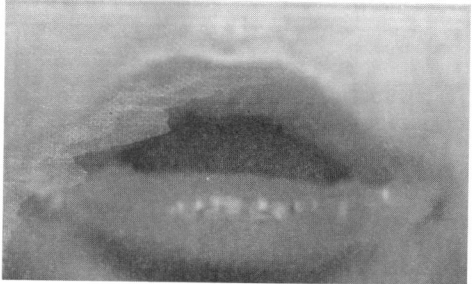

Exhibit 4.1 Angular stomatitis

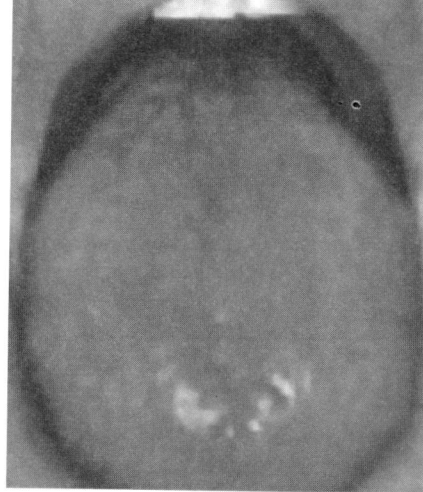

Exhibit 4.3 Glossitis

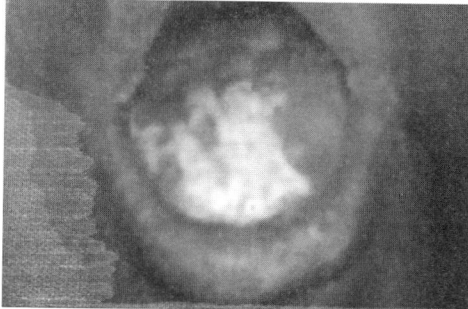

Exhibit 4.2 Candidal infections

3. **Identify the clinical condition from the photograph.**

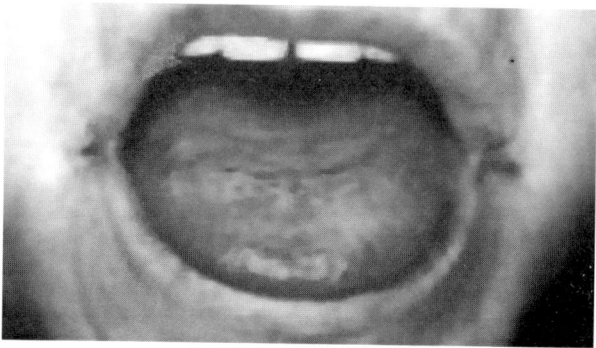

Exhibit 4.4 Angular cheilitis

Ans. It is angular cheilitis due to riboflavin deficiency.

HISTORICAL ASPECT

Jan Jacbz Swammerdam (1637–1680)

He was a biologist and microscopist. As part of his anatomical research, he carried out experiments on contraction of muscle. In 1658, he was the first to observe and describe the RBC. He was one of the first people to use the microscope in dissections, and his techniques remained useful for hundreds of years.

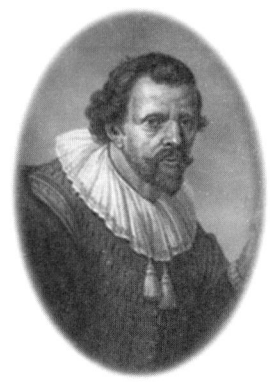

Jan Jacbz Swammerdam

RECENT UPDATES

The hematologic conditions associated with orofacial signs and symptoms include mainly sickle cell anemia, iron deficiency anemia, megaloblastic anemia and thalassemia. The oral manifestation in hematologic diseases may manifest as atrophic glossitis, dysphagia, angular stomatitis, post-extraction bleeding and gingival bleeding. The patient may also present with osteosclerosis, osteomyelitis, and paraesthesia/anesthesia within the trigeminal system. The sickle cell anemia patients at times experience severe facial pain associated with blood vessel occlusion. Aplastic anemia patients are susceptible to oral ulceration, fungal infection and viral infection. In practice one should be careful while prescribing drugs for dental ailment in patients with hematological diseases. Aspirin or non-steroidal medication should be avoided in patient of anemia with acid peptic disorders. The sickle cell anemia patient should only be given dental treatment when they are not in the crisis. The anti-fungal medications are prescribed as part of treatment in iron-deficiency anemia patients manifesting with angular cheilitis and candidiasis.

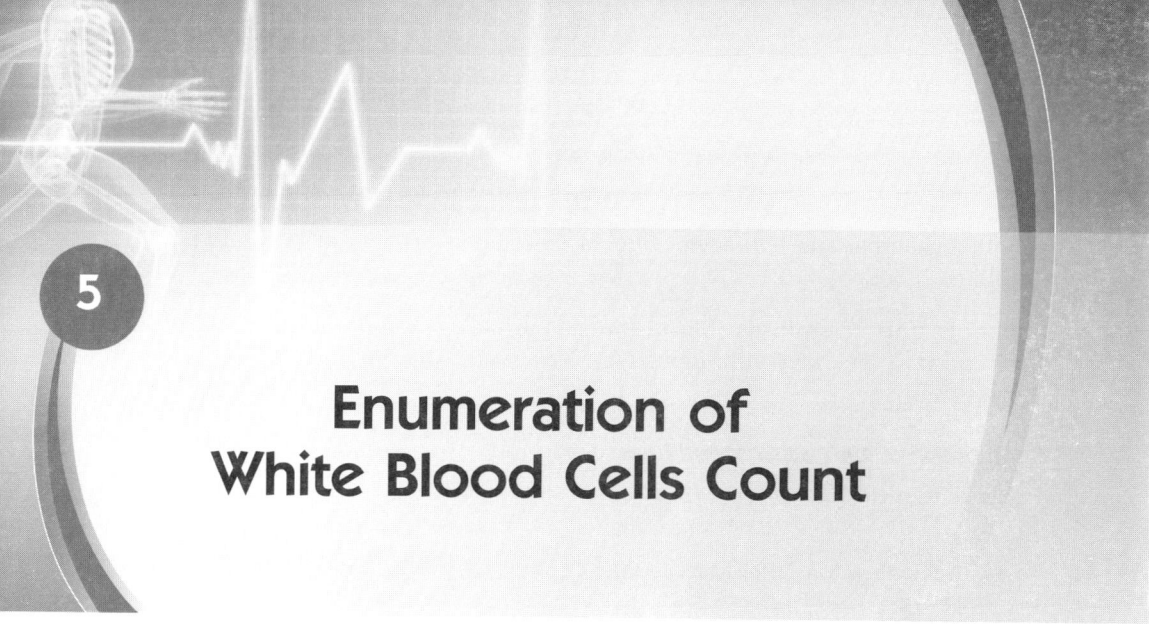

Enumeration of White Blood Cells Count

Learning Objectives

After learning this practicals, the student should be able to:

1. Carry the total leukocyte count by the manual method and report the observed value of the total white blood cell (WBC) count.
2. Describe the normal and altered total leukocyte count in physiological and pathological conditions.
3. Describe the functions and regulation of leukopoiesis.

INTRODUCTION

Leukocyte provides immunity against pathogens and thus helps in defending off disease. The normal WBC count in adults ranges between 4000/cu mm and 11000/cu mm. The count after birth is around 18000/cu mm to 20000/cu mm which returns to physiological levels in a few years time. The count increases in physiological conditions such as heavy exercise, stress, pregnancy, menstruation, etc.

DENTAL PERSPECTIVE

Decrease in leukocyte is seen in infection with nonpyogenic organisms, viral infections and protozoal infections. When such patients report for oral diseases or treatment, it should be remembered that such patients are at high risk for further getting bacterial infections; especially one should be careful while monitoring patients of gum diseases, thrush, deep mouth sores and mouth ulcers.

Aim: Determine the total leukocyte count (TLC) in 1 cu mm of blood.

Principle: The blood sample is diluted with a diluting fluid which destroys the red cells and stains the nuclei of the leukocytes. The cells are then counted in a counting chamber and leukocyte count is reported as number of WBCs in 1 cu mm of undiluted blood.

Materials and chemicals: Blood lanced/pricking needle, sterile cotton swabs, spirit, microscope, coverslip, hemocytometer, WBC pipette and WBC diluting fluid (Turk's fluid).

Composition of WBC diluting fluid (Turk's fluid)

- Glacial acetic acid: 3 mL (hemolyze RBCs)
- Gentian violet: 1 mL of 1% (stain the nuclei of the WBCs)
- Distilled water (to make up to 100 mL).

Procedures

1. Take 1 mL of Turk's fluid in a watch glass. Keep the counting chamber on the microscope stage and focus the 16 WBC squares.
2. Give a sterile finger prick and wipe away the first drop of blood. Wait till free flow of blood is there and then draw blood into the pipette up to the 0.5 mark.
3. The tip of the pipette is to be wiped with gauze piece and then draw the Turk's fluid up to the 11 mark. Gently mix the blood and diluting fluid in the bulb.
4. Wait for 10 minutes for the lysis of the RBC.
5. After discarding the first two drops charge the Neubauer's chamber and wait for 2 minutes for the cells to settle.
6. Check for even distribution of cells in the four corner squares under the low power objective.
7. Count the total number of WBCs in the four corner squares using the low power objective.

Calculation

- Area of the four WBC squares = 4 × 1 = 4 sq mm.
- Depth under the coverslip (distance between coverslip and glass of Neubauer's chamber) = 1/10 mm. Therefore, volume of fluid in four WBC square = 4 × 1/10 = 4/10 cu mm.
- The number of WBCs in 4/10 cu mm of diluted blood = n cells.
- The number of WBCs in 1 cu mm of diluted blood = n × 10/4 cells.
- The dilution factor = 1:20 (0.5 parts of blood in 10 parts of Turk's fluid). Therefore, the number of WBCs in 1 cu mm of undiluted blood.

$= n \times 10/4 \times 20/1$

$= n \times 50$ cells.

Results: Record your observation and result:

The WBC count is _____.

DENTAL IMPLICATION

Total leukocyte count is done as routine before any dental procedure or surgery. Leukocyte counts are altered in periodontal diseases and facial cellulitis because of the invasion by the bacterial pathogens. Facial cellulitis of odontogenic origin causes a characteristic alteration in the white cell count of the blood. The specific findings are neutrophilia, monocytosis, eosinopenia, basopenia and generalized leukocytosis. If patients have neutropenia they are more likely to get infections. If there are not enough neutrophils, the inflammatory changes are absent (redness or swelling along the infection site). This means infections, such as periodontal (gum) disease, yeast infections and oral ulcers, can get worse quickly. People with severe neutropenia can have deep ulcers (sores) in their mouths. These sores are often painful.

OBJECTIVE STRUCTURED PRACTICAL EXAMINATION (OSPE) QUESTIONS

Draw the blood from given sample in WBC pipette.

Student 1

1. Draw blood into the WBC pipette up to 0.5 mark. (Yes/No)
2. The tip of the pipette is wiped with gauze piece and the Turk's fluid is drawn up to 11 mark. The blood is mixed gently in the bulb. (Yes/No)

Charge the Neubauer's chamber

Student 2

1. Discard the first two drops and then charge the Neubauer's chamber and wait for 2 minutes for the cells to settle. (Yes/No)
2. Check for even distribution of cells in the four corner squares under the low power objective. (Yes/No)

VIVA QUESTIONS

1. **What is the function of the bead in white cell pipette bulb?**

Ans. The bead in white cell pipette bulb aids mixing the blood with the diluents, informs whether the pipette is dry or not and helps in identifying the pipette.

2. **What are the uses of WBC pipette?**

Ans. The WBC pipette can be used for counting WBC, RBC, platelets and counting sperms.

3. **Where does hematopoiesis occur?**

Ans. Hematopoiesis occurs in the bone marrow (mainly within flat bones, where erythrocytes, leukocytes and platelets are formed) and in the lymphoid tissue (site for the maturation of leukocytes) of the thymus, spleen and lymph nodes.

4. **What are the types of leukocytes and how are they classified into granulocytes and agranulocytes?**

Ans. The types of leukocytes are lymphocytes, monocytes, neutrophils, eosinophils and basophils. The neutrophils, eosinophils and basophils are granulocytes in whose cytoplasm have granules (when viewed under electronic microscopy). Agranulocytes are lymphocytes and monocytes.

5. **What is the generic function of leukocytes? What leads to leukocytosis and leukopenia?**

Ans. The generic function of leukocytes is to actively participate in the defense of the body against pathogens.

Leukocytosis: It is due to increase in the number of WBCs beyond 11,000/mm irrespective of the type of cells (granulocytes, monocytes, lymphocytes, etc).

(a) Physiological leukocytes are seen in normal infants, after intake of food and after digestion, physical exercise, pregnancy, mental stress, parturition, etc.

(b) Pathological leukocytosis is seen in acute pyogenic bacterial infection (Streptococcus, Staphylococcus), myocardial infarction, acute hemorrhage, burns, malignancies or postsurgical postoperative rise.

Leukopenia: It is a decrease in the number of white cells below the normal lower limit of 4,000/cu mm.

(a) Physiological leukopenia is rare and marginal decrease may be seen in extreme cold conditions as in arctic environment exposure.

(b) Pathological leukopenia are seen in:
- Infection with nonpyogenic organisms (typhoid and paratyphoid fevers, protozoal infection like malaria, etc)
- Viral infections (influenza, mumps, smallpox and acquired immuno-deficiency syndrome)
- Drugs (chloramphenicol, sulphonamides, aspirin, penicillins, phenytoin, etc)
- Repeated exposures to X-rays and radium during radiotherapy in cancers
- Malnutrition (deficiency of vitamin B and folate, etc)

MULTIPLE CHOICE QUESTIONS

1. **The normal WBC count is:**

   A. 4,000–6,000

   B. 6,000–7,100

   C. 4,000–11,000

   D. 2,000–3,000

2. **The pathological cause of leukocytosis is:**

   A. Pyogenic infection

   B. Stress

   C. Pregnancy

   D. Exercise

3. **The ratio of WBC and RBC is:**
   A. 1:6
   B. 1:60
   C. 1:600
   D. 1:6,000

4. **The most abundant granulocyte in human blood is:**
   A. Neutrophil
   B. Basophil
   C. Eosinophil
   D. None of the above

5. **Which of the following organs is most essential for proper immune maturation and functioning:**
   A. Spleen
   B. Liver
   C. Thyroid
   D. Thymus

6. **WBCs squeeze through pores in capillary wall by:**
   A. Chemotaxis
   B. Diapedesis
   C. Pinocytosis
   D. Opsonization

7. **Which of the following are not phagocytes?**
   A. Dust cells
   B. Eosinophils
   C. Microglia
   D. Plasma cells

8. **Regarding granulopoiesis, which statement is not true?**
   A. Duration is 2 weeks
   B. Occurs exclusively in red bone marrow
   C. Wholly extravascular process
   D. Dead granulocytes play an important role in its regulation

9. **Which of the following do not belong to others?**
   A. Eosinophil
   B. Basophil
   C. Histocyte
   D. Neutrophil

Answers:

1 C	2 A	3 C	4 D	5 B	6 B	7 D	8 A
9 C							

CLINICAL CASE SCENARIO

1. **How shall you treat a patient with decreased total leukocyte count reported to you for dental ailment?**

Ans. The patient's complete medical history needs to be evaluated with confirmation of his/her complete blood cell count. If he/she is suffering from anemia or having decreased leukocyte count, his/her clinical condition and diagnosis should be confirmed with consultation of patient's physician. Precautionary measures are to be followed prior as dental procedures are being carried out in patients having decreased WBC count or in patients of aplastic anemia by prescribing antibiotics coverage as well as use an antibiotic mouthwash. If your patient is having chronic anemia, you should be ready with oxygen during certain procedures. If your patient has disorders that would lead to uncontrolled bleeding, you may also use antifibrinolytic medications. You may also need to take additional precautions based on the type of procedure, and the current condition of the blood count.

HISTORICAL ASPECT

Gabriel Andral (1797–1876)

Gabriel Andral was a distinguished French pathologist and a Professor at the University of Paris. He was the founder of the science of hematology and integrated science into clinical and investigative medicine. He was also the first physician to assess the potential of chemical analysis of the blood.

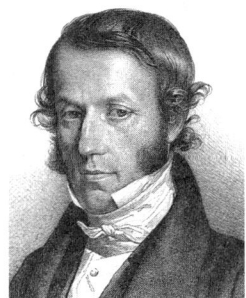

In the year 1843, Gabriel Andral, a French professor of medicine and William Addison, a British physician, simultaneously discovered WBC. They believed that both red and white cells were altered in disease.

Gabriel Andral

RECENT UPDATES

A new class of WBCs was discovered by the scientist in the year 2013 in human lung and gut tissues. They play a critical role as the first line of defense against harmful bacterial and fungal infections. This will help scientists to design better targeted vaccine strategies to treat cancer and infections such as hepatitis B. The immune responses against infectious agents are activated and regulated by dendritic cells (DCs). The dendritic cells are a specialized group of WBCs which present tiny fragments from microorganisms, vaccines or tumors to the T cells. T helper 17 (Th17) cells play a key role in activating a protective response crucial for our body to eliminate harmful bacteria or fungi. In this study, the scientists identified a new subset of DCs (named CD11b + DCs) which are capable of activating such protective Th17 response.

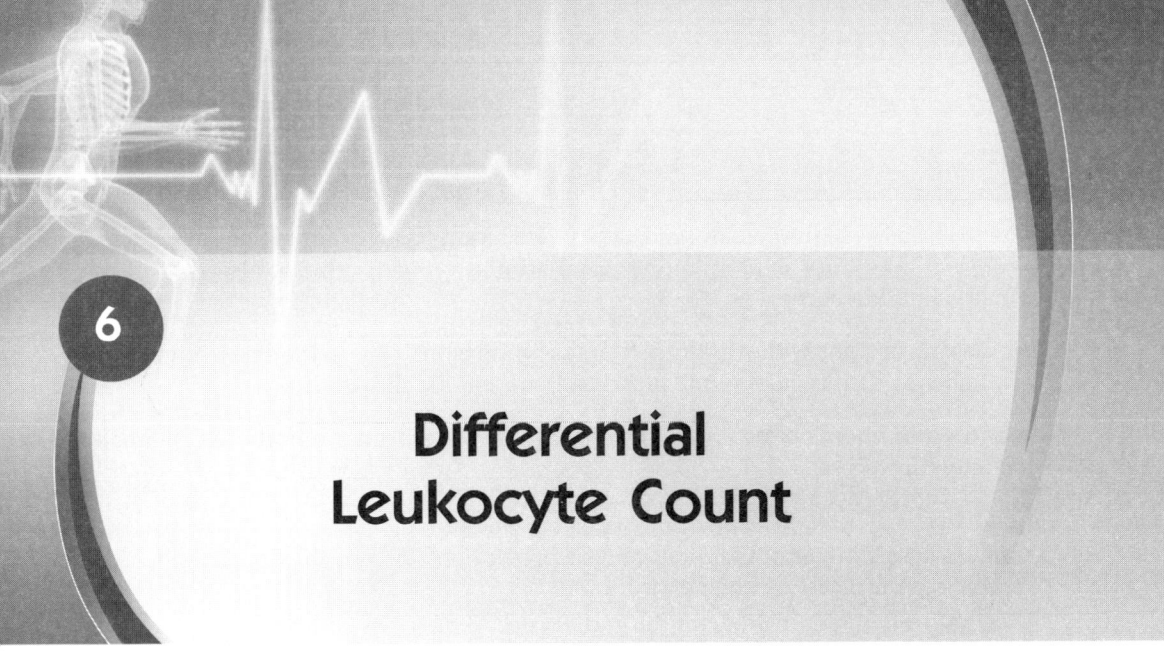

Differential Leukocyte Count

Learning Objectives

After completing the practicals, the student should be able to:

1. Make an ideal smear and stain the slide for differential leukocyte count.
2. Identify the neutrophil, eosinophil, basophil, monocyte and lymphocyte in smear slide.
3. Determine the number of each type of white blood cell present in the blood and expressed them as a percentage of each type among the total hundred cell counted.

INTRODUCTION

White blood cells are the cell of defense to combat against bacterial and viral infection in the human body. The normal count in adults ranges between 4000/cu mm and 11000/cu mm. As on the basis of its morphological appearance under a light microscope and tinctorial characteristics when stained; leukocytes are divided into five classes of leukocytes: Neutrophils (40–75%), eosinophils (1–6%), basophils (less than 1%), monocytes (2–10%) and lymphocytes (20–45%).

Collectively, neutrophils, eosinophils, and basophils are known as granulocytes due to the presence of granules in their cytoplasm. In addition, monocytes and lymphocytes are also known as mononuclear cells.

DENTAL PERSPECTIVE

The complete blood count including WBC and DLC are immensely helpful for making diagnostic, prognostic and therapeutic advices. The use of the complete blood count by dentists has been limited and most complete blood count examinations are ordered as routine laboratory examinations upon admission to the hospital for operative dentistry and oral surgery.

Aim: To stain and study the different types of white blood cells in the smear. Determine the number of each type of white blood cell, present in the blood.

Materials and chemicals: Lancet, clean dry glass slides, cedar wood oil, Leishman's stain and microscope.

Procedures
1. Make a sterile finger prick under aseptic precaution. Discard the first drop of blood and allow the blood to free flow.
2. Place a drop of blood at one of the end of each of the glass slides.
3. Place the spreader slide at an angle of 45° just in front of the blood drop.
4. Move the spreader slide backward to touch the blood drop.
5. The drop must spread out along the line of contact of the spreader slide.
6. Move the spreader slide smoothly and evenly in forward direction maintaining an angle of 45° to make the blood smear.
7. Let the smear dry in air. Repeat the procedure and make three more blood smears.

> (**Note:** An ideal smear is uniform without any striations or vacuoles and neither too thin nor too thick.) A smear is described as having a head, body and tail.

Fixing of blood slide: The smear is being fixed by adding acetone free methyl alcohol. The slide is kept covered with acetone free methyl alcohol for a minute. Alcohol denatures the proteins and hardens the cell contents.

Stain preparation and staining: The composition of Leishman's stain contains 0.15 gm powdered Leishman's stain and 133 mL of methyl alcohol. Leishman's stain belongs to the Romanowsky group of stains. It is a mixture of methylene blue and eosin in acetone free methyl alcohol. Methylene blue which is a basic dye stains cytoplasm, nucleus and granules of basophils. Eosin is an acidic dye which stains the granules of the eosinophils and RBCs. Acetone free methyl alcohol is a fixative. It causes precipitation of the proteins thus aiding the blood smear to get fixed to the slide and is prevented from being washed off.

Method of staining: Pour a few drops of Leishman's stain on the slide so as to cover it under the stain and wait for 2 minutes. Add adequate amount of buffered water. Mix by rocking and wait for 7–10 minutes. The stain is flooded off with distilled water so as to clear any overstained portion and then allow it to dry.

Examination of a blood film
• The dry and stained film is examined without a cover slip under oil immersion objective. Place a drop of cedar wood oil over the chosen area and move the oil immersion objective into position; making the lower end of the objective touch the drop of oil.

- Focus the cell using fine adjustment knob. The differential cell count is done by moving the slide along the central and periphery of the smear. A total of 100 cells are to be counted in which every white cell seen must be recorded as neutrophil, basophil, eosinophil, monocyte and lymphocyte.

PRECAUTIONS

1. Clean and dry the slides before use.
2. The glass-spreader must have a smooth and clean edge for uniform spreading of the blood drop.
3. Prepare 2–3 slides at a time for practice and obtain an ideal smear.
4. Well-stained slide should be examined under the oil-immersion lens for appropriate results.

   Then find the percentage of each type.

Results

N = _____%,   E = _____%,

B = _____%,   L = _____%,

M = _____%

DENTAL IMPLICATION

Though differential leukocyte count (DLC) is done as routine before any dental procedure or surgery, but it has significant impact in periodontal disease and facial cellulitis. Facial cellulitis of odontogenic origin causes a characteristic alteration in the white cell count of the blood. The specific findings are neutrophilia, monocytosis, eosinopenia, basopenia and generalized leukocytosis.

Systemic inflammatory responses to periodontal bacteria have been suggested as a pathogenetic link between periodontal disease and atherosclerosis. Many risk factors that might contribute to the pathogenesis of atherosclerosis have been proposed including chronic inflammation and infection. Levels of WBCs and platelets are elevated in periodontitis patients suggesting chronic inflammation and infection as predisposing cause of atherosclerosis in periodontics.

OBJECTIVE STRUCTURED PRACTICAL EXAMINATION (OSPE) QUESTIONS

Prepare a Blood Smear

1. Place a drop of blood at one of the end of each of the glass slides.   (Yes/No)
2. Place the spreader slide at an angle of 45° just in front of the blood   (Yes/No)
   drop.

3. Move the spreader slide backward to touch the blood drop.   (Yes/No)

4. The drop must spread out along the line of contact of the spreader   (Yes/No)
slide.

5. Move the spreader slide smoothly and evenly in forward direction   (Yes/No)
maintaining an angle of 45° to make the blood smear.

VIVA QUESTIONS

1. **Tabulate the types of white blood cell as per size and the characteristic of their nucleus and cytoplasm.**

Ans. The types of white blood cell as per size and the characteristic of their nucleus and cytoplasm are:

Cell type	Size (micron)	Nucleus	Cytoplasmic granules
Neutrophil	12–14	Multilobed	Fine violet pink granules
Eosinophil	12–14	Bilobed	Coarse brick red granules
Basophil	12–14	2–3 lobes	Coarse bluish black granules
Monocyte	14–21	Round, oval or kidney shape	Fine azurophilic granules (not seen in light microscopy)
Lymphocyte large	12–14	Round	Agranular
Lymphocyte small	8–10	Round	Agranular

2. **Identify the cells.**

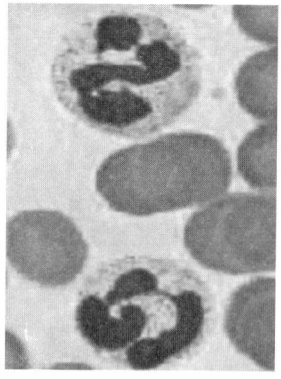

Exhibit 6.1 Neutrophil

Ans. Neutrophil

3. **Identify the cells.**

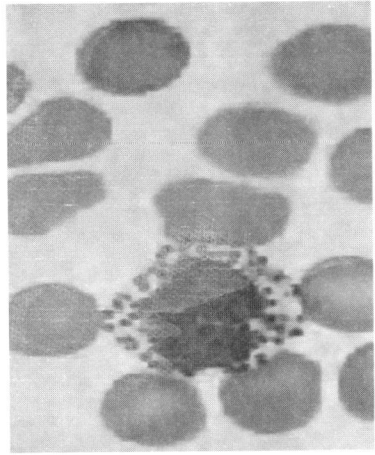

Exhibit 6.2 Eosinophil

Ans. Eosinophil

4. **Identify the cell.**

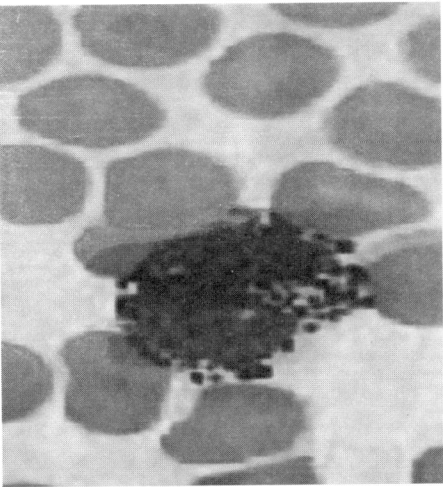

Exhibit 6.3 Basophil

Ans. Basophil (bilobed nucleus and dark purple granules are seen in allergies and parasitic infections).

5. **Identify the cells.**

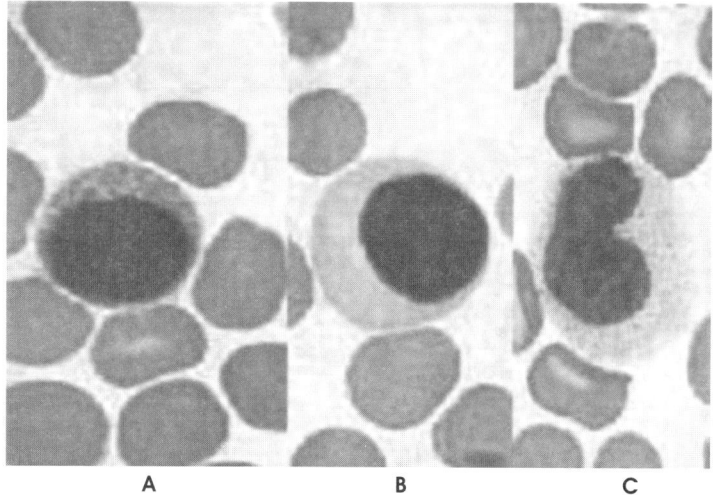

A   B   C

Exhibit 6.4 (A and B) Lymphocyte and **(C)** Monocyte

Ans. A and B are lymphocyte and C is monocyte.

6. **Enlist the causes for decreased and increased neutrophil count.**

Ans. The neutrophil count is decreased in: **Congenital causes**—hereditary neutropenia, and **acquired**—bone marrow disease, immune reactions, drugs (phenothiazenes, benzodiazepines, antithyroids, anticonvulsants, quinine, quinidine, indomethacin, procainamide, thiazides, etc), Gram-negative septicemia and myeloproliferative disorders.

The neutrophil count is increased in pregnancy, after exercise, after injection of epinephrine, in pyogenic infections and following tissue destruction (burns, hemorrhage, etc).

7. **Enlist the causes for decreased and increased eosinophil count.**

Ans. Eosinopenia (decrease in eosinophil count) seen after injection of ACTH or after corticosteroids therapy. Eosinophilia (increase in eosinophil count) seen in allergic conditions like bronchial asthma, allergic dermatitis and parasitic infections.

8. **Enlist the causes for lymphocytosis and lymphopenia.**

Ans. Lymphocytosis (increase in lymphocytes) is seen in children (normal count is 40–60%), lymphocytic leukemia, viral infection and in chronic infections like tuberculosis.

Lymphopenia (decrease in lymphocytes) is seen in hypoplastic bone marrow and acquired immune deficiency syndrome.

9. **Enlist the causes for monocytosis and monocytopenia.**

Ans. Monocytosis (increase in monocytes) seen in tuberculosis, syphilis and some leukemias.

Monocytopenia (decrease in monocytes) seen in hypoplastic bone marrow.

10. Discuss the genesis of granulocytes and agranulocytes from blood stem cell.

Ans. The genesis of granulocytes and agranulocytes from its precursor is as follows:

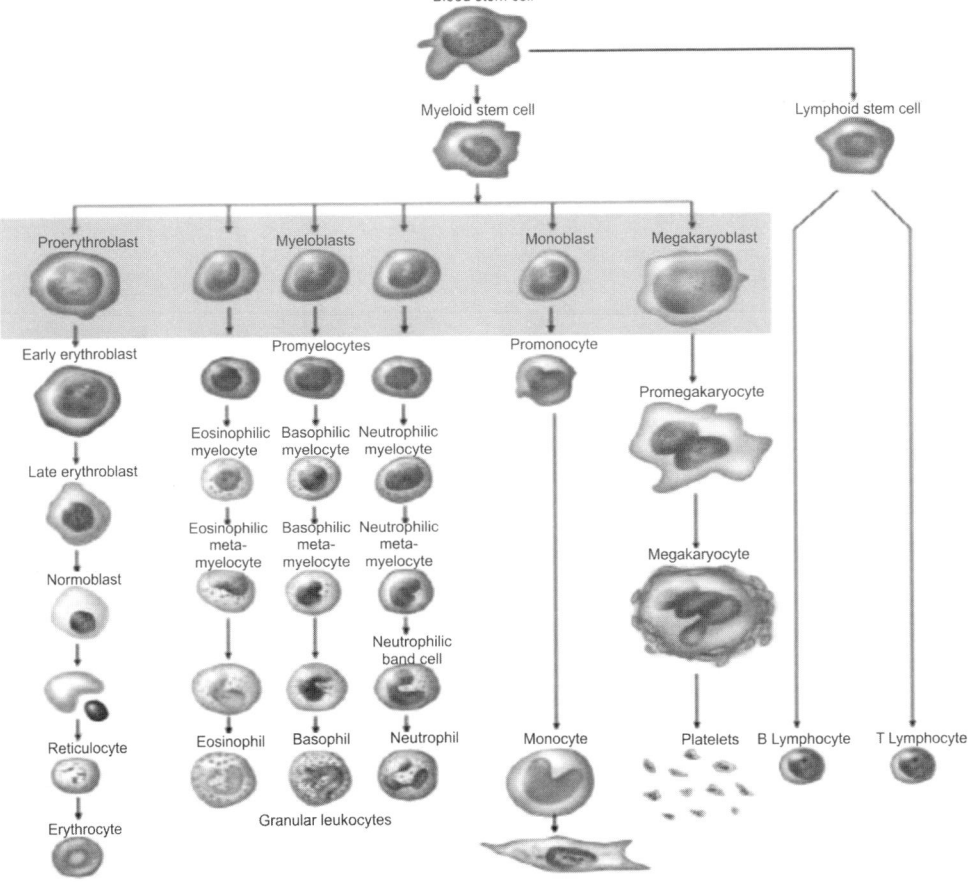

Fig. 6.1 Genesis of granulocytes and agranulocytes from blood stem cells.

MULTIPLE CHOICE QUESTIONS

1. The granules of neutrophil are:
    A. Fine numerous pink in color
    B. Fine numerous green in color
    C. Fine numerous blue in color
    D. Fine numerous red-brown in color

2. **The granules of eosinophil are:**
   A. Large coarse brick red in color
   B. Large coarse green in color
   C. Large coarse orange in color
   D. Fine numerous purple in color

3. **The granules of basophil are:**
   A. Coarse red in color
   B. Coarse purple/blue in color
   C. Coarse green in color
   D. Coarse pink in color

4. **The normal size of small and large lymphocyte is:**
   A. Small: 2–4 micron and large: 1–4 micron
   B. Small: 7–10 micron and large: 10–14 micron
   C. Small: 4–6 micron and large: 6–8 micron
   D. Small: 17–22 micron and large: 30–44 micron

5. **The normal percentage of monocyte is:**
   A. 2–4%
   B. 0–1%
   C. 3–4%
   D. 2–8%

Answers:				
1 D	2 A	3 B	4 B	5 D

CLINICAL CASE SCENARIO

1. **The increase in white blood cell count (WBC) and platelet count due to systemic inflammation and infection is considered a risk factor for cardiovascular diseases. These parameters increase in periodontal disease. How can the WBC count and platelet count be reverted to physiological level? What is its advantage?**

Ans. A decrease in WBC and platelet counts by periodontal therapy may decrease the risk for cardiovascular disease. Periodontal therapy reduces the TLC and platelet count, thereby possibly decreasing the risk for the development of cardiovascular disease by lowering the established risk factors for periodontal atherosclerosis.

HISTORICAL ASPECT

Paul Ehrlich (1854–1915)

He was a German Jewish physician and scientist who worked in the field of hematology, immunology and chemotherapy. He invented the precursor technique to Gram-staining bacteria, and his methods of staining tissue made it possible to distinguish between different types of blood cells, and this helped to diagnose numerous blood diseases. Ehrlich used both alkaline and acid dyes, and also created new, "neutral" dyes. For the first time, this made it possible to differentiate the lymphocytes among the leukocytes (white blood cells). He stained their granulation and could distinguish between nongranular lymphocytes, mononuclear and polynuclear leukocytes, eosinophil granulocytes and mast cells.

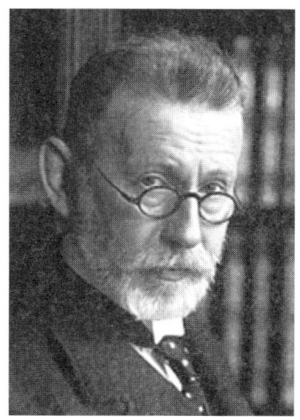

Paul Ehrlich

RECENT UPDATES

Digital morphology is immensely helpful in pressing operational, quality, and patient care needs in clinical hematology laboratory nowadays. The manual WBC differential otherwise time consuming can now be improved in terms of performance time, accuracy and consistency. The clinician can view all cells on a single computer screen; they can make immediate assessments of whether or not a sample is abnormal enough to warrant closer inspection. The system confirms the cell counter's results and flags if necessary. This confirmation process may take about a minute rather than the average of 5–6 minutes currently being spent. The tasks of sending slide for a pathologist's review are now eliminated altogether because the images can be saved in a database and can be accessed remotely and in real-time by the pathologist.

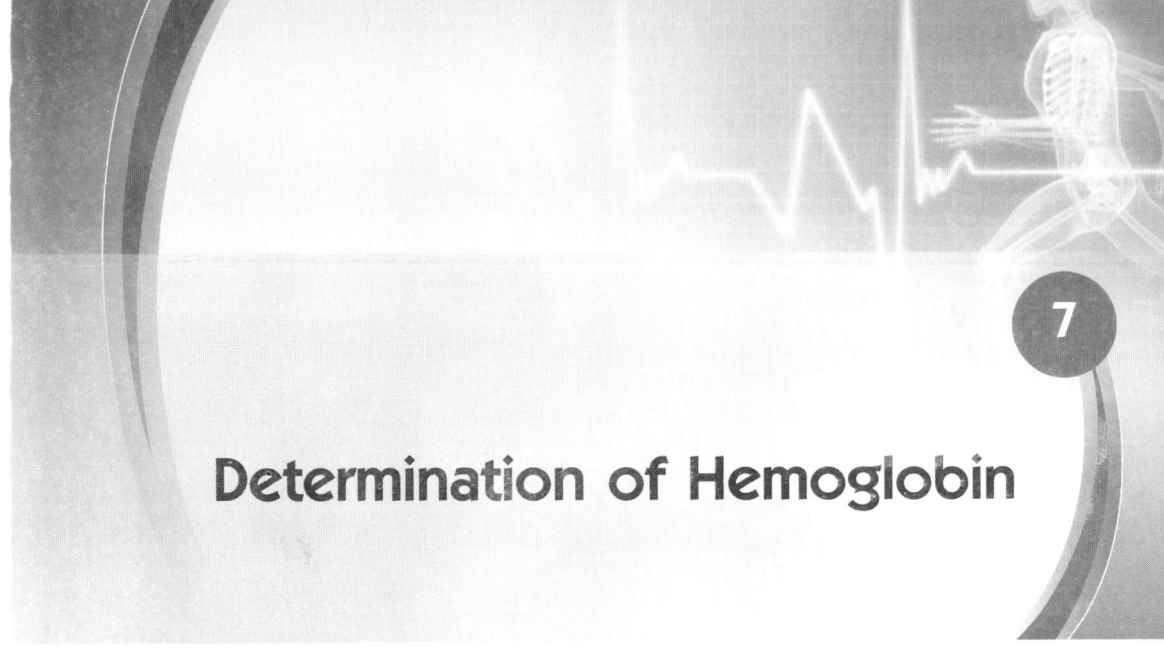

Determination of Hemoglobin

> **Learning Objectives**
> After completion of practicals, the student should be able to:
> 1. Estimate the hemoglobin using Shali's method.
> 2. Discuss the other methods for estimation of hemoglobin.
> 3. Enlist various clinical conditions in which the hemoglobin concentration is altered.

INTRODUCTION

Hemoglobin estimation is done routine in clinical setup to rule out anemia. The other common causes of low hemoglobin include loss of blood (traumatic injury, surgery, bleeding from colonic or gastric carcinoma, etc), nutritional deficiency (iron, vitamin B_{12} and folate), bone marrow problems (replacement of bone marrow by cancer), suppression by chemotherapy drugs, kidney failure, or abnormal hemoglobin structure (sickle-cell anemia and thalassemia).

Numbers of methods are available for hemoglobin (Hb) estimation amongst which Sahli's method for testing hemoglobin is one of the most acceptable visual methods.

DENTAL PERSPECTIVE

Hemoglobin estimation is routinely recommended in patients in whom signs of anemia are visible and so also prior to any dental procedures or surgery. Some of the oral effects seen in patient of anemia are increased risk for periodontitis, gum diseases or glossitis. As the procedure is easy to perform, the patient's hemoglobin concentration can be done in dental clinic or along the bedside before starting any dental procedures.

Aim: Estimation of the hemoglobin concentration.

Sahli's Acid Hematin Method

Principle

The Hb present in blood is converted by addition of dilute hydrochloric acid into acid hematin. Acid hematin appears golden brown in color. The observed golden brown color depends on the concentration of Hb. The color of the solution is matched against golden brown-tinted glass color of the comparator. The hemoglobinometer tube is graduated on one side in gram percent (gm%) from 2 to 24, and on the other side, as percentage (%) from 20 to 140. The Hb concentration for the value when the color of solution matches with comparator is noted in gm%.

Apparatus

1. Sahli's hemoglobinometer contains a comparator, hemoglobin tube, hemoglobin pipette and stirrer.

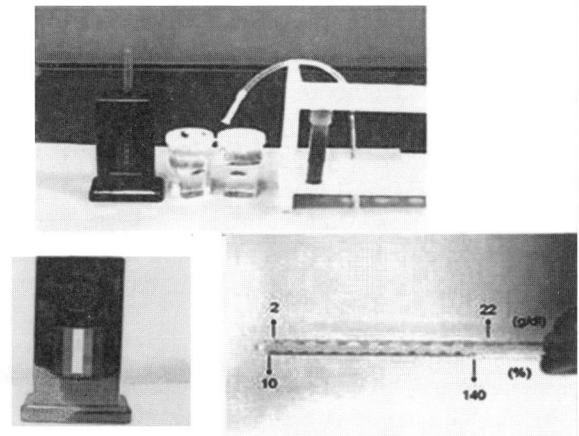

Acid hematin method (Sahli's method)

Fig. 7.1 Sahli's hemoglobinometer

Hemoglobin tube: It is graduated on one side in gm% from 2 to 24 and on the other side as percentage from 20 to 140. This tube is called Sahli-Adams tube.

Comparator: The hemoglobin tube is accommodated in middle slot. The nonfading standard brown-tinted glass pieces are provided on either side of the slot for the color matching. The opaque white glass fitted at the back provides uniform illumination.

Hemoglobin pipette: The pipette bears a mark indicating 20 cu mm (0.2 mL). The bulb is not available in the pipette.

Stirrer: It is a thin glass rod which is used for stirring the solution.

2. N/10 HCL

3. Distilled water

4. **Dropper:** Ordinary glass dropper or Pasteur pipette which is an 8–10 inch glass tube with a long thin nozzle and its rubber teat is used as dropper.
5. **Materials for a sterile finger prick:** Sterile lancet, sterile gauze, cotton swabs and methylated spirit.

Procedures

1. Ensure that hemoglobinometer tube and pipette are clean and dry.
2. Add N/10 HCL in the hemoglobinometer tube up to its lowest mark (10% or 2 g%) with the help of a dropper.
3. Clean the finger with methylated spirit using the cotton gauze and prick the finger under all aseptic precautions. Discard the first drop of blood.
4. Allow a large drop of blood to form on the fingertip, and then dip and draw blood up to 20 cu mm mark of the pipette.
5. Wipe the tip of the pipette and transfer 0.02 mL of blood from the pipette into the hemoglobinometer tube containing N/10 HCL by immersing tip of the pipette in the acid solution and blowing out blood from the pipette.
6. Leave the solution in the hemoglobinometer tube for about 10 minutes (for conversion of hemoglobin to acid hematin which occurs in the first 10 minutes).
7. Dilute the acid hematin by adding distilled water drop by drop. Mix it with the stirrer. Match the color of the solution in the hemoglobinometer tube with the standards of the comparator. After addition of every drop of distilled water, the solution should be mixed and the color of the solution should be compared with the standard of the comparator till it matches with that of the standard. Take care to hold the stirrer above the level of the solution. At no stage should the stirrer be taken out of the tube.
8. Note the reading when the color of the solution exactly matches with the standard and express the hemoglobin content as gm%.

PRECAUTIONS

1. All aseptic precaution should be used during pricking.
2. The first drop of blood should be discarded and do not squeeze the finger because tissue fluids which comes out gives lower values of hemoglobin.
3. Wait for at least 10 minutes for the formation of acid hematin by the action of hydrochloric acid on Hb.
4. Avoid over dilution as later the color cannot be concentrated.
5. Golden brown color of the solution should be compared with the standard of the comparator till it matches with that of the standard of the comparator.
6. Take care to hold the stirrer above the level of the solution. At no stage should the stirrer be taken out of the tube.

Advantages and disadvantages of Sahli's acid hematin method

The advantages are: Sahli's hemoglobin meter is portable, easy to carry anywhere (bedside in case of critical patient, outpatient department (OPD) in hospital at field visit during clinical studies, etc) and it is easy to perform and handle.

Disadvantages

(a) The standard coloration on the hemoglobinometer fades away over the year and this will give wrong result.

(b) It gives results in approximation only and not accurately and cannot be fully relied upon.

Results

1. Hb concentration in the provided subject is _____.
2. 1 gm of hemoglobin carries 1.34 mL of oxygen, hence the oxygen carrying capacity in the subject is _____.

Normal values

1. Adult males: 14–18 (16.2) g/dL of blood
2. Adult females: 12–16 (14.2) g/dL of blood.

DENTAL IMPLICATION

Some of the oral effects which may manifest in patient of anemia are:

• Increased risk for periodontitis or gum disease.

• Inflammation of the tongue leads to glossitis and tongue may appear swollen, smooth and pale, and it may feel sore and tender.

Oral Manifestations in Iron Deficiency Anemia

This anemia is mainly caused due to inadequate dietary intake of iron, faulty absorption of iron and increased requirement for iron. The Plummer-Vinson syndrome is a form of anemia with iron deficiency, dysphagia, kolinichia and atrophic glossitis.

Iron deficiency anemia manifests as cracks or fissure at the corners of mouth, a lemon tinted pallor of skin, smooth, red painful tongue with atrophy of filiform papilla, fungiform papilla and dysphagia. The mucous membrane appears pale with signs of glossitis and angular stomatitis.

Oral Manifestations: Thalassemia

An unusual prominence of the premaxilla, pale oral mucosa and maxillary teeth are irregularly arranged. Intraoral radiograph shows peculiar trabecular pattern of maxilla, coarsening of trabecula and blurring.

Disappearance of other resulting "salt and pepper effect" thickening of diploe of skull. Inner and outer plates become elongated producing bristles like crew cut or hair on end appearance.

Oral Manifestations: Sickle Cell Anemia

Oral manifestation is mainly on radiographic findings where marrow spaces are remarkably enlarged because of loss of many trabeculae. Osteoclastic area appears as noted hair on end appearance on skull.

OBJECTIVE STRUCTURED PRACTICAL EXAMINATION (OSPE) QUESTIONS

OSPE I

1. Ensure hemoglobinometer tube and pipette are clean and dry. (Yes/No)

2. Add N/10 HCL in the hemoglobinometer tube up to its lowest (Yes/No)
   mark (10 per cent or 2 g%) with the help of a dropper.

3. Draw blood up to 20 cu mm mark of the pipette from the given (Yes/No)
   sample.

4. Wipe the tip of the pipette and transfer the 0.02 mL of blood from (Yes/No)
   the pipette into the hemoglobinometer tube containing N/10 HCL
   by immersing tip of the pipette in the acid solution and blowing
   out blood from the pipette.

5. Leave the solution in the hemoglobinometer tube for about (Yes/No)
   10 minutes (for conversion of hemoglobin to acid hematin
   which occurs in the first 10 minutes).

> The student should leave the tube in the comparator for acid hematin formation. The technician will take care of further step.

OSPE II

> A technician after waiting for 10 minutes has kept the hemoglobinometer tube ready. Golden brown color of acid hematin is visible.

1. Dilute the acid hematin by adding distilled water drop by drop. (Yes/No)
   Mix it with the stirrer. Match the color of the solution in the hemoglobinometer tube with the standards of the comparator.

2. After addition of every drop of distilled water, the solution should (Yes/No)
   be mixed and the color of the solution should be compared with the
   standard of the comparator till it matches with that of the standard.

3. Take care to hold the stirrer above the level of the solution. At no (Yes/No)
   stage should the stirrer be taken out of the tube.

4. Note the reading when the color of the solution exactly matches (Yes/No)
   with the standard and express the hemoglobin content as gm%.

VIVA QUESTIONS

1. **Enlist the various methods of estimation of hemoglobin concentration.**

Ans. Hemoglobin can be estimated by various methods and categorically can be classified as:

   (i) Visual methods include Sahli's method, Wintrobes method, Haldanes method and Tallquists method

   (ii) Gasometric method includes cyanmethemoglobin method, Van Slyke method, spectrophotometric method and oxyhemoglobin method

   (iii) Automated hemoglobinometry

   (iv) Other methods include alkaline hematin method, specific gravity method and comparator method.

2. **Discuss the various methods of estimation of hemoglobin.**

Ans. The various methods of estimation of hemoglobin are:

   A. **Spectrophotometric method:** These methods are rapid and give accurate results.

   (i) *Oxyhemoglobin method:* Ammonium hydroxide (0.04 mL/dL) which is used to hemolyze the red cells convert the hemoglobin to oxyhemoglobin which is measured in the spectrophotometer. This conversion is immediate and the resulting color is stable.

   (ii) *Cyanmethemoglobin method:* The best recommended method is the cyanmethemoglobin method. In this method, blood is diluted in a solution containing potassium cyanide and potassium ferri-cyanide (Drabkin's solution), Hb is oxidized to methemoglobin by potassium ferri-cyanide, methemoglobin in turn combines with potassium cyanide to form cyanmethemoglobin. The absorbance of the solution is measured in a spectrophotometer at wavelength 540 nm against Drabkin's solution as a blank (standard). Hemoglobin values are calculated from a hemoglobin curve using a hemoglobin standard.

   B. **Gasometric method:** Gasometric method of estimation of hemoglobin is by using Van Slyke apparatus. This method is not used routinely in clinical laboratories as it is time consuming and the process of estimation is complex.

   C. **Automated hemoglobinometry:** Various automated techniques have been employed to measure hemoglobin.

   D. **Specific gravity method:** This method uses the principle that when a drop of whole blood is dropped into a solution of copper sulfate, which has a given specific gravity, the drop will maintain its own density for approximately 15 seconds. The density of the drop is directly proportional to the amount of hemoglobin in that drop.

   E. **Comparator method:** This is a visual method and diluent used is an alkali solution (ammonia solution 0.04%). After mixing with dilute ammonia solution, the intensity of the color of the hemolyzed solution of red blood cells is compared against a standard color disk in the comparator.

F. **Tallquist method:** The method involves direct matching of the red color of a drop of whole fresh blood on a filter paper with color standards on the paper. Depending on the color hemoglobin concentration value as depicted in the standard is noted as result.

G. **Haldane method:** In this method, hemolysis of red cells is produced by mixing blood with the hypotonic solution; like distilled water. Carbon monoxide is added to the mixture. The color of the solution is compared with the standard one.

3. **What are the functions of hemoglobin?**

Ans. **The functions of hemoglobin are:** Hemoglobin transports oxygen from the lungs to the tissues, and carbon dioxide from the tissues to the lungs and also acts as a buffer in maintaining blood pH.

4. **What is the name of the molecule that transports oxygen in red blood cells?**

Ans. The respiratory pigment of the red blood cells is hemoglobin.

5. **What is the molecular composition of hemoglobin? Does the functionality of hemoglobin as a protein depend upon its tertiary or upon its quaternary structure?**

Ans. Hemoglobin is a molecule made of four polypeptide chains, each bound to an iron-containing molecular group called a heme group. So, the molecule contains four polypeptide chains and four heme groups.

   As a protein composed of association of polypeptide chains, the functionality of hemoglobin depends upon the integrity of its quaternary structure.

6. **What are the types of hemoglobin and its variant?**

Ans. The types of hemoglobin and its variant are:

In the embryo:
- Gower 1 ($\zeta_2\varepsilon_2$)
- Gower 2 ($\alpha_2\varepsilon_2$)
- Hemoglobin Portland I ($\zeta_2\gamma_2$)
- Hemoglobin Portland II ($\zeta_2\beta_2$).

In the fetus:
- Hemoglobin F ($\alpha_2\gamma_2$)

In adults:
- **Hemoglobin A ($\alpha_2\beta_2$):** The most common with a normal amount over 95%.
- **Hemoglobin A$_2$ ($\alpha_2\delta_2$):** δ chain synthesis begins late in the third trimester and in adults, it has a normal range of 1.5–3.5%.
- **Hemoglobin F ($\alpha_2\gamma_2$):** In adults hemoglobin F is restricted to a limited population of red cells called F-cells. However, the level of HbF can be elevated in persons with sickle cell disease and beta thalassemia.

Variant forms that cause disease:
- **Hemoglobin H (β_4):** It may be present in variants of α thalassemia.
- **Hemoglobin Bart's (γ_4):** A variant form of hemoglobin, formed by a tetramer of γ chains, which may be present in variants of α thalassemia.
- **Hemoglobin S ($\alpha_2\beta_2^S$):** A variant form of hemoglobin found in people with sickle cell disease.
- **Hemoglobin C ($\alpha_2\beta_2^C$):** Another variant due to a variation in the β-chain gene. This variant causes a mild chronic hemolytic anemia.
- **Hemoglobin E ($\alpha_2\beta_2^E$):** Another variant due to a variation in the β-chain gene. This variant causes a mild chronic hemolytic anaemia.
- **Hemoglobin AS:** A heterozygous form causing sickle-cell trait with one adult gene and one sickle cell disease gene.

7. **What is the molecular weight of hemoglobin?**

Ans. Hemoglobin is a globular molecule having a molecular weight of 68,000.

8. **What is the normal blood hemoglobin level in adult male and adult female?**

Ans. The normal hemoglobin concentration in adult male is 15.5 g/dL (range 14–18 g/dL) and in female it is 14 g/dL (range 12–15.5 g/dL).

9. **What is the normal hemoglobin concentration at birth and 1 year of age?**

Ans. At birth the concentration of hemoglobin increases and may reach up to 23 g/dL. It occurs due to:
   (a) hemoconcentration by reduction in plasma volume and
   (b) transfusion of cells from placenta to infant.
      After 2 days of birth the HB level starts decreasing and stabilizes at the end of 3 months to 10. 5 g/dL. At 1 year of age the Hb concentration rises to 12 g/dL.

10. **Hb concentration of a given subject was found to be 14 gm%, calculate its oxygen carrying capacity percentage.**

Ans. The normal hemoglobin carrying capacity of blood per gram of hemoglobin is 1.34 mL; hence the oxygen carrying capacity of the subject is $14 \times 1.34 = 18.76$ mL/dL.

11. **Enlist the normal variant of hemoglobin.**

Ans. (a) Normal adult hemoglobin (HbA), hemoglobin A2 (HbA2)
   (b) Fetal hemoglobin (HbAF).

12. **What are the advantages and disadvantages of Sahli's method?**

Ans. **Advantages of Sahli's method:** Sahli's hemoglobin meter is portable, easy to carry anywhere (bedside in case of critical patient, OPD in hospital, field visit during clinical studies, etc) and it is easy to perform and handle.

Disadvantages of Sahli's method:
   (a) The standard coloration on the hemoglobinometer fades away over the year and this will give wrong result.
   (b) It gives results in approximation only and not accurately and cannot be fully relied upon.

8. **What is the function of N/HCL?**

Ans. Hydrochloric acid acts with hemoglobin to form acid hematin. The brown color which appears when the reaction is complete and quantative and can be compared with color of comparator as standard matching.

9. **What is the principle of Hb estimation?**

Ans. In this method, Hb is converted to acid hematin CN-10 HCL. The brownish yellow color of the solution is matched with color of a standard comparator to give rough estimate of Hb in gm%.

10. **Which is most accurate method of Hb estimation?**

Ans. Cyanmethemoglobin method is most accurate because estimation is done with photoelectric colorimeter.

11. **Define anemia. Grade the severity of anemia based on hemoglobin values.**

Ans. (a) Mild anemia: Hemoglobin 8–12 gm%
(b) Moderate anemia: Hemoglobin 5–8 gm%
(c) Severe anemia: Hemoglobin 5 gm%.

MULTIPLE CHOICE QUESTIONS

1. **The heme is an iron porphyrin complex called:**
   A. Iron-protoporphyrin VII
   B. Iron-protoporphyrin IX
   C. Iron-protoporphyrin X
   D. Iron-protoporphyrin XI

2. **The iron in heme is in:**
   A. Ferrous (Fe^{2+}) form   B. Nitrous form
   C. Sulphurous form   D. Potash form

3. **Life span of HBF is around:**
   A. 2–3 weeks   B. 1–2 weeks
   C. 3–4 weeks   D. 4–6 weeks

4. **Heme is synthesized in:**
   A. Golgi complex   B. Ribosomes
   C. Lysosomes   D. Mitochondria

5 **Sickle-shaped cells:**
   A. Decreases blood viscosity, thereby decreasing blood flow to the tissue
   B. Increases blood viscosity, thereby decreasing flow to the tissue
   C. Increases blood viscosity, thereby increasing blood flow to the tissue
   D. Blood viscosity remain unaltered

6. One hemoglobin molecules contain _____ iron atoms.
   A. 8   B. 4
   C. 2   D. 1

7. The affinity of hemoglobin is _____ times for carbon monoxide than oxygen:
   A. 20   B. 50
   C. 250   D. 125

8. Hemoglobin combines with oxygen to form:
   A. Oxidation   B. Oxygenation
   C. Oxyhemoglobin   D. Deoxyhemoglobin

9. Adult hemoglobin has_____chains.
   A. 2 alpha, 2 beta   B. 2 alpha, 2 delta
   C. 3 alpha   D. 6 alpha

10. Beta-thalassemia minor:
    A. HBF level remains unchanged
    B. HBF level is markedly increased
    C. HBF level is markedly decreased
    D. HBF chains are absent

11. Hemoglobin's iron content is:
    A. 2%   B. 3%
    C. 0.33%   D. 4%

12. The commonest form of thalassemia is:
    A. Beta minor   B. Beta major
    C. Alpha   D. Beta

13. On completion of life span of RBC hemoglobin is degraded into amino acid which is:
    A. Excreted in urine
    B. Excreted in stool
    C. Joins the amino acid pool of plasma
    D. Secreted in bile

14. Reduced hemoglobin is:
    A. Deoxygenated hemoglobin   B. Corbamino hemoglobin
    C. Oxyhemoglobin   D. Methemoglobin

Answers:

1 B	2 A	3 B	4 D	5 B	6 B	7 C	8 C
9 A	10 B	11 C	12 A	13 C	14 A		

CLINICAL CASE SCENARIO

Case 1

A 35-year-old patient came with history of fissure at the corners of mouth, red painful tongue and complaints difficulty in chewing and swallowing. His hemoglobin level was 10 gm% and peripheral smear showed microcytic hypochromic anemia.

1. **What is your diagnosis? Discuss the clinical manifestation in the diseased condition.**

Ans. The patient is suffering from atrophic glossitis due to iron deficiency anemia. Difficulty in swallowing is due to atrophy of filiform papilla and fungiform papilla. The patient may present with dysphagia, glossitis, blurring of the tongue and angular stomatitis. The patient is treated with iron supplementation and advice intake of diet rich in iron.

Self Study

Case 2

2. **Study the radiological findings in patient of thalassemia major.**

Ans. The oral manifestations of thalassemia major includes mucosal pallor and dental malocclusion in particular, which can be a useful pointer to prompt the clinician to suspect this disorder in undiagnosed cases.

The prevalence of dental complications which are observed in β-thalassemia major patients: Loss of trabecular pattern, thinning of lamina dura and hair-on-end appearance of skull.

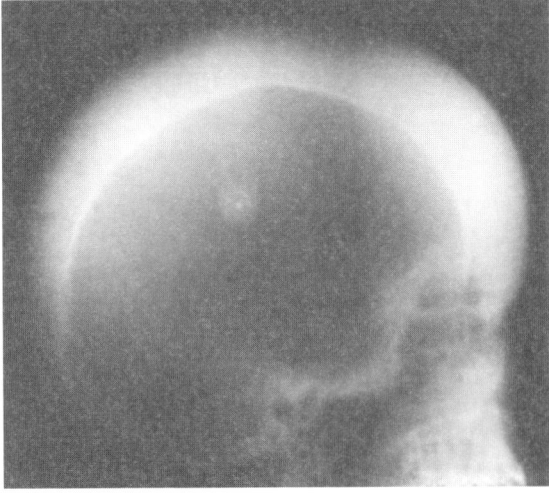

Exhibit 7.1 Hair-on-end appearance of skull

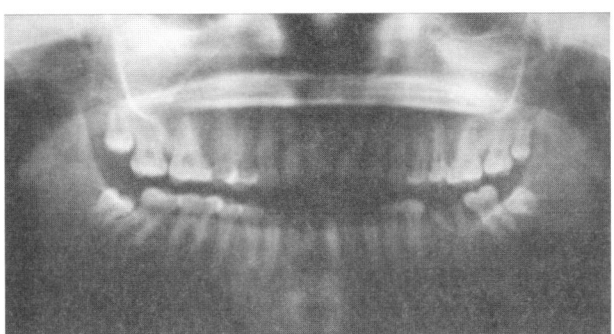

Exhibit 7.2 Thinning of lamina dura and loss of trabecular pattern

β-thalassemia major patients may also present with malocclusion and proclination of teeth.

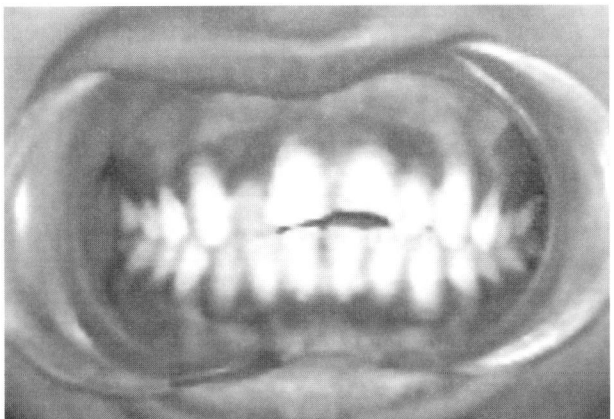

Exhibit 7.3 Malocclusion of teeth

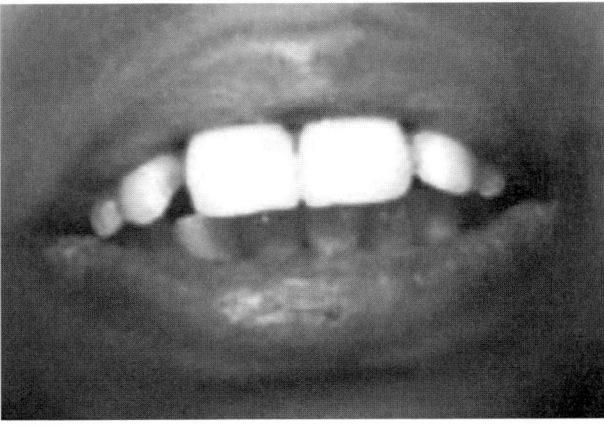

Exhibit 7.4 Proclination of teeth

Case 3

History: A 29-year-old Indian man referred for consultation due to pain in his lower teeth. Patient has a history of inflammatory bowel disease. Family history revealed that his father had sickle cell trait. The patient came to the dental clinic with X-ray film and hydroxyurea tablet in his pocket.

The radiological finding suggested changes in bone density of lower jaw and hair-on-end appearance on skull and the intraoral examination revealed pale mucus membrane with swelling. Noting the clinical, oral and radiological findings.

3. What disease is patient suffering from?

Ans. The patient is suffering from sickle cell anemia. This may be confirmed by hemoglobin electrophoresis and sickling test.

HISTORICAL ASPECT

Max Perutz
(19 May 1914–6 February 2002)

His Triumph: The structure of hemoglobin.

Perutz's main contribution was to work out the structure of hemoglobin, the large molecule that carries oxygen through the blood, for which he shared the Nobel Prize for Chemistry in 1962.

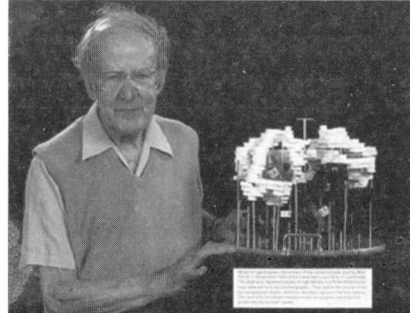

Max Perutz

James Herrick
(11 August 1861–7 March 1954)

The first clinical description of sickle cell disease.

In 1910, James Herrick described the presence of elongated and sickle-shaped red blood corpuscles; in a blood sample of a 20-year-old dentistry student from Grenada. In recounting his observation in the Archives of Internal Medicine, Herrick provided the first clinical description of sickle-cell disease in the western medical literature.

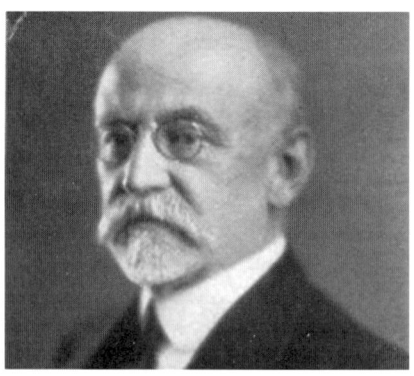

James Herrick

Thomas Benton Cooley
(23 June 1871–13 October 1945)

He was an American pediatrician and hematologist and professor of hygiene and medicine at the University of Michigan and Wayne State University.

He made the first definitive description of thalassemia in 1925 along with his collaborator Pearl Lee. Cooley gained acclaim for his scientific work in the field of pediatric hematology and is principally remembered for his discovery of, and research into, a form of childhood anemia that became known as Cooley's anemia.

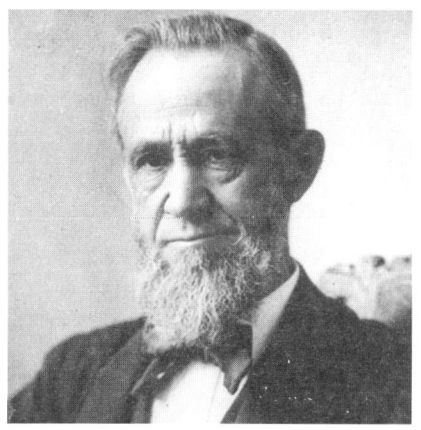

Thomas Benton Cooley

RECENT UPDATES

A. Glycated hemoglobin (HbA1c) is usually a reliable indicator of diabetic control. Chromatography of normal adult blood divides into two parts:

1. HbA (HbA0): 92–94%.
2. HbA1 (6–8%) where the B chain has an additional glucose group.

HbA1 itself consists of three different glycations, the HbA1c subgroup being the most useful, usually measured by isoelectric focusing or electrophoresis.

The glycation of hemoglobin occurs at a variable (nonlinear rate) over time during the whole life span of the red blood cell (RBC) which is normally 120 days. This means the relative proportion of glycated hemoglobin at any one time depends on the mean glucose level over the previous 120 days.

Normal levels (laboratory normal "range") will differ depending on whether HbA1 or HbA1c is measured, and the method used—use your laboratory's reference range [EDTA (FBC) bottle].

B. A hemoglobin electrophoresis test is a blood test done to check the different types of hemoglobin in the blood.

The most common types of normal hemoglobin are:

- *Hemoglobin F (fetal hemoglobin):* This type is normally found in fetuses and newborn babies. Some diseases, such as sickle-cell diseases, aplastic anemia and leukemia have abnormal types of hemoglobin and higher amount of hemoglobin F.
- *Hemoglobin A:* This is the most common type of hemoglobin found normally in adults.
- *Hemoglobin A2:* This is a normal type of hemoglobin found in small amount in adults.

More than 400 different types of abnormal hemoglobin have been found, but the most common are:

- *Hemoglobin S:* This type of hemoglobin is present in sickle cell disease.
- *Hemoglobin C:* This type of hemoglobin does not carry oxygen well.
- *Hemoglobin E:* This type of hemoglobin is found in people of Southeast Asian descent.
- *Hemoglobin D:* This type of hemoglobin is present in sickle cell disease.
- *Hemoglobin H (heavy hemoglobin):* This type of hemoglobin may be present in certain types of thalassemia.
- *Hemoglobin S and C* are the most common types of abnormal hemoglobins that may be found by an electrophoresis test.

Electrophoresis uses an electrical current to separate normal and abnormal types of hemoglobin in the blood. Hemoglobin types have different electrical charges and move at different speeds. The amount of each hemoglobin type in the current is measured.

An abnormal amount of normal hemoglobin or an abnormal type of hemoglobin in the blood may mean that a disease is present. For example, hemoglobin S is found in sickle cell disease.

Hemoglobin electrophoresis is done to find type of hemoglobin in the blood. This can be used to diagnose certain types of anemia (such as thalassemia).

8

Determination of Blood Groups (A, B, O and Rh System)

Learning Objectives

The learner after completing practical should be able to:

1. Determine the blood group using anti-A, anti-B and anti-D.
2. Describe the indications of blood transfusion.
3. Explain the hazards of mismatched blood transfusion.
4. Enlist the precautions while carrying blood grouping.

INTRODUCTION

Blood group stands as an important identity tag of an individual and mentioned in working identity card and driving license. Blood grouping is essential for record prior

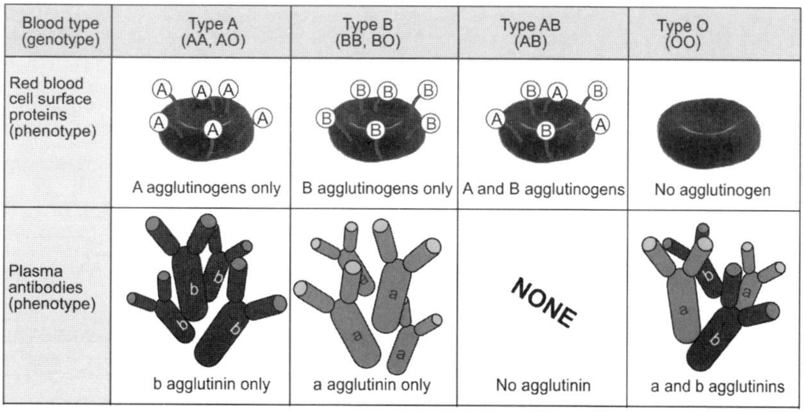

Blood type (genotype)	Type A (AA, AO)	Type B (BB, BO)	Type AB (AB)	Type O (OO)
Red blood cell surface proteins (phenotype)	A agglutinogens only	B agglutinogens only	A and B agglutinogens	No agglutinogen
Plasma antibodies (phenotype)	b agglutinin only	a agglutinin only	No agglutinin	a and b agglutinins

Fig. 8.1 Blood genotypes of the ABO blood group system

to any dental procedures and surgery. The blood group is identified by the antigens present on red blood cells which react with antibodies which are added as antisera A, B and D and agglutination is observed. These antigens are called agglutinogens and antibodies which develop against the antigens are agglutinins. There are around 32 known blood group systems out of which ABO and Rh systems are important. ABO system has A and B antibodies in individual from birth with corresponding antigen being absent in the individual. Based on the experiment they are classified as blood group A, B, AB and O.

RH SYSTEM

Rh antigens also known as D antigens are transmembrane proteins with loops exposed at the surface of red blood cells. Rh antigen when present on red cell membrane of an individual, the blood group is Rh D positive; if not, it is Rh D negative. They appear to be used for the transport of carbon dioxide and/or ammonia across the plasma membrane. They are named for the rhesus monkey in which they were first discovered. Eighty-five percent of the population is Rh D positive, the other 15% of the population have Rh D negative blood.

DENTAL PERSPECTIVE

The dental invasive procedures and oral surgery have risk of bleeding in their patients. The need of blood transfusion may arrive during surgery. Blood group must be recorded during routine dental check-up as a precautionary measure.

Principle: Blood group determination is done by using specific agglutinins (antibodies) to confirm the presence or absence of the corresponding agglutinogen (antigen) on the RBC membrane.

METHOD

Apparatus and materials: Anti-A serum, anti-B serum, anti-D, test tubes, slides, 0.9% saline.

Preparation of a red cell suspension:
- Take 2 mL of isotonic 0.9% saline in a clean test tube.
- The finger should be pricked under aseptic conditions till free flow of blood is obtained and wipe away the first drop of blood.
- Add the next drop of blood to the saline in the tube by inverting the tube over drop of blood so as to make a red cell suspension.
- Do not add a drop of blood directly to the anti-A or anti-B serum as it can give false positive results.

Determination of the blood group: Take three clean glass slides and mark them as follows with a glass marking pencil.

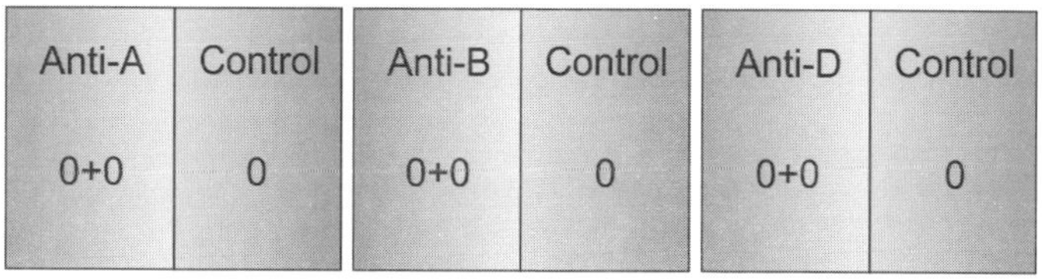

Anti-A	Control	Anti-B	Control	Anti-D	Control
0+0	0	0+0	0	0+0	0

Fig. 8.2 Glass slide with antisera A, B and D

• Place a drop of corresponding antiserum-A, (i.e. serum containing antibodies A), antiserum-B (serum containing B-antibodies) and antiserum Rh (serum containing antibodies, anti-D) at the prior noted spots with the help of a dropper. In addition, one drop of isotonic saline (used as control) is also placed on each slide which acts as control.

• The red cell suspension is drawn from the bottom of the test tube into capillary dropper and a drop of it is added to each of the divisions on the glass slides.

• Mix the antisera and red cell suspension with separate applicator rod.

• After waiting for 10 minutes, gently rock the slide back and forth.

• Observe for the agglutination and confirm your finding under the low power of the microscope (RBCs are clumped together and lose their outline).

• Compare it with the saline controls. In control, the RBCs remain separated and evenly distributed.

• Record the presence (+)/absence (–) of agglutination.

Table 8.1 Agglutination pattern of ABO blood groups

Anti-A serum	Anti-B serum	Agglutinogens	Blood group
+	–	A	A
–	+	B	B
+	+	A, B	AB
–	–	Neither	O

Interpret the results as above.

(**Note:** False positive reaction can occur due to use of antisera contaminated with bacterial growth or due to loss of potency of the antisera because of improper storage.)

PRECAUTIONS

1. The slides should be cleaned and dried.
2. Aseptic precaution should be followed while pricking and the finger should not be squeezed for obtaining blood drop. The prick should be bold and blood allowed to free flow.

3. The slide should be labeled before placing the antisera A, B and Rh and isotonic saline.
4. Examine the slide for agglutination before the solution dries up. The findings should be confirmed under the low power of the microscope.

DENTAL IMPLICATION

The blood type and manifestation of particular diseases cannot be made a dictum but many researchers have tried to evaluate the incidence of various diseases and observed correlation with the blood types.

Periodontal disease: Research studies repeatedly show distinct differences between the blood types and the rates of occurrence of periodontal disease and gingivitis. The research findings in a few studies concluded that type A and type B individuals have higher occurrence rate of periodontal disease and gingivitis than type O individual. The people who are type A, type B, and type AB are able to secrete A, B (or A and B) antigens in their saliva, in addition to the O or H antigen.

Dental caries: There are a few research studies on blood type and dental caries (cavities) stating that the blood group A individuals may have lower levels of cavities than the other blood groups, especially if the group A subjects were secretors.

Periodontal disease versus dental caries: It has been noted from literature that many groups with high rates of caries have low rates of periodontal disease and vice versa. This may be true of blood groups as well. Type O has been known to have lower frequencies of periodontal disease perhaps because they carry both anti-A and anti-B antibodies, thus being protected again more strains of periodontitis—causing bacteria than A, B or AB.

VIVA QUESTIONS

1. **Discuss the clinical application of blood grouping.**

Ans. The blood grouping is useful for:
   (a) Safe blood transfusion
   (b) Preventing hemolytic disease
   (c) Resolving paternity disputes
   (d) Arriving at conclusion in medicolegal cases
   (e) Knowing susceptibility to diseases

2. **Name the methods for detection of antigen–antibody reaction serologically.**

Ans. The antigen–antibody reactions in blood group serology are usually detected by haem-agglutination, complement fixation, neutralization, absorption, elution and precipitation.

3. **Which methods and procedures can be used in performing blood grouping?**

Ans. Three manual methods that can be used when performing blood grouping are glass slide or white porcelain tile method, glass test tube method and microwell plate method. The newer techniques are column technique (sephadex gel) and solid phase tests.

4. **Name the various blood group systems.**

Ans. Apart from ABO and Rh systems, there are 30 group systems that have been identified. In addition to the ABO antigens and Rh antigens, many other antigens are expressed on the RBC surface membrane. For example, an individual can be AB, D positive, and at the same time M and N positive (MNS system), K positive (Kell system), Le^a or Le^b negative (Lewis system) and likewise being positive or negative for each blood group system antigen. These blood group systems were named after the patients in whom the corresponding antibodies were initially encountered.

5. **Discuss the hazards of blood transfusion.**

Ans. Hazards of mismatched blood transfusion are:

1. Mismatched transfusion reactions include agglutination, tissue ischemia, hemolysis of agglutinated red cells occur rapidly releasing a large amount of hemoglobin in circulation, hemolytic jaundice, renal vasoconstriction caused by toxic substances released from the hemolyzed RBCs, circulatory shock, hemoglobinuria, renal tubular damage, acute renal shut down (anuria) and uremia.

2. Circulatory overload due to hypervolemia.

3. Transmission of blood-borne infections such as AIDS, viral hepatitis, malaria, syphilis, etc.

4. Pyrogenic reactions

5. Allergic reactions

6. Hyperkalemia

7. Hypocalcemia.

6. **If an Rh negative mother carries Rh positive fetus, discuss the likely complications.**

Ans. When an Rh negative mother carries Rh positive fetus, RBCs containing D-antigen may enter the maternal circulation at the time of delivery. The mother shall form anti-D and during second pregnancy, the antibodies will enter the fetal circulation and tend to destroy fetal red blood cell causing hemolytic disease of the newborn.

7. **Enlist the various forms of clinical manifestation of hemolytic disease of the newborn.**

Ans. The various forms of clinical manifestation of hemolytic disease of the newborn are:

   (i) Hydrops fetalis

   (ii) Icterus gravis neonatorum (hemolytic jaundice)

   (iii) Kernicterus

   (iv) Erythroblastosis fetalis.

8. **Describe the Landsteiner's law.**

Ans. The Landsteiner's law states that if an agglutinogen is present on red cell membrane, the corresponding agglutinin may be absent in the plasma. If agglutinogen is not present on red cell membrane, the corresponding agglutinin will be present in plasma. The second half of the definition is not applicable to all blood groups. For example, in Rh negative individual the absence of agglutinogen on red cell membrane is not accompanied by presence of agglutinin in plasma.

9. **Why ABO incompatibilities rarely produce hemolytic disease of the newborn?**

Ans. ABO incompatibilities are rare because A and B antibodies are of IgM type and cannot cross the placenta.

10. **Which safety procedures should be followed to prevent blood transfusion complication?**

Ans. Direct cross matching of the blood is the only safeguard against blood transfusion complication. It involves matching the serum of the recipient directly against the RBCs of the donor (major cross matching) and again to match the RBCs of the recipient against the serum of the donor (major cross matching).

11. **What will happen if individual is transfused with an incompatible blood group?**

Ans. If an individual is transfused with an incompatible blood group, destruction of the red blood cells will occur and this may result in the death of the recipient mainly due to disseminated intravascular coagulation.

MULTIPLE CHOICE QUESTIONS

1. **Which of the following is essential for blood clotting?**

   A. RBC   **B.** WBC

   C. Blood platelets   **D.** Lymph

2. **During blood coagulation, thromboplastin is released by:**

   A. Red blood cell

   B. Blood plasma

   C. Leukocytes

   D. Clumped platelets and damaged

3. **ABO blood type antigens are found:**

   A. At the surface of red cells   **B.** Saliva

   C. Tears and urine   **D.** All of the above

4. _____ **was awarded the Nobel Prize in Physiology or Medicine in 1930 for his discovery of blood types:**

   A. Adolf Creite   **B.** Thomas Young

   C. Leonard Landois   **D.** Karl Landsteiner

5. **Major cross matching involves:**
   A. Matching the serum of the recipient directly against the RBCs of the donor
   B. Matching the RBCs of the recipient directly against the serum of the donor
   C. Matching the WBCs of the recipient directly against the serum of the donor
   D. Matching the RBCs of the recipient directly against the saliva of the donor

6. **The antigens present in an individual of blood group A are:**
   A. A antigens
   B. B antigens
   C. AB antigens
   D. C antigens

7. **The hemolytic disease of newborn is:**
   A. Erythroblastosis fetalis
   B. Addison's disease
   C. Cushing syndrome
   D. Graves' disease

8. **Which of the following elements shows a little change in stored blood?**
   A. Potassium   **B.** Sodium
   C. Calcium   **D.** Magnesium

9. **Half-life of platelet is:**
   A. 4 hours   **B.** 12 hours
   C. 21 hours   **D.** 24 hours

Answers:

1 C	2 D	3 D	4 D	5 A	6 B	7 A	8 B
9 B							

HISTORICAL ASPECT

Karl Landsteiner (1868–1943)

Karl Landsteiner discovered that blood clumping was an immunological reaction which occurs when the receiver of a blood transfusion has antibodies against the donor blood cells.

Karl Landsteiner's work made it possible to determine blood types and thus paved the way for blood transfusions to be carried out safely. For this discovery, he was awarded the Nobel Prize in Physiology or Medicine in 1930.

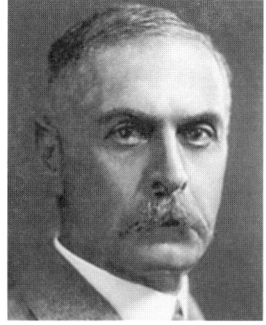

Karl Landsteiner

Leonard Landois (1837–1902)

He was born 1837 in Münster. A medical student at the University of Greifswald and later Professor and Director of the Institute of Physiology at Greifswald studied blood transfusions and the phenomena of agglutination. In 1875, he published work titled "Die Transfusion des Blutes". He died 1902 in Greifswald.

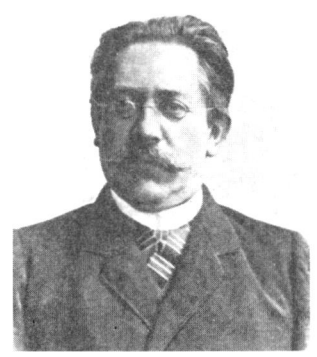

Leonard Landois

RECENT UPDATES

There are 308 blood group determinants and more than 30 known blood group system. Bombay blood group which was first discovered in Bombay is also known as h/h or Oh blood group. This is a rare blood type and it has resulted due to mutation that leads to deficiency of H antigen. The H antigen is the precursor of O antigen. This blood type is characterized by the absence of O, A and B antigens and is observed in 1 in 250,000 individuals worldwide. A weaker expression of H antigen has also been identified and the blood group is known as para-Bombay blood group.

9

Determination of Bleeding Time and Clotting Time

INTRODUCTION

Blood coagulation refers to the process of forming of a clot which arrest bleeding. Three mechanism involved in clotting are vasoconstriction, platelet plug formation and platelet clot formation.

The clotting cascade occurs through two separate pathways that interact: (1) the intrinsic and (2) the extrinsic pathways.

Extrinsic pathway: The extrinsic pathway is activated by external trauma that causes blood to escape from the vascular system. This pathway is quicker than the intrinsic pathway. It involves factor VII.

Intrinsic pathway: The intrinsic pathway is activated by trauma inside the vascular system, and is activated by platelets, exposed endothelium, chemicals or collagen. This pathway is slower than the extrinsic pathway, but more important. It involves factors XII, XI, IX, VIII.

Common pathway: Both pathways meet and finish the pathway of clot production in what is known as the common pathway. The common pathway involves factors I, II, V, and X.

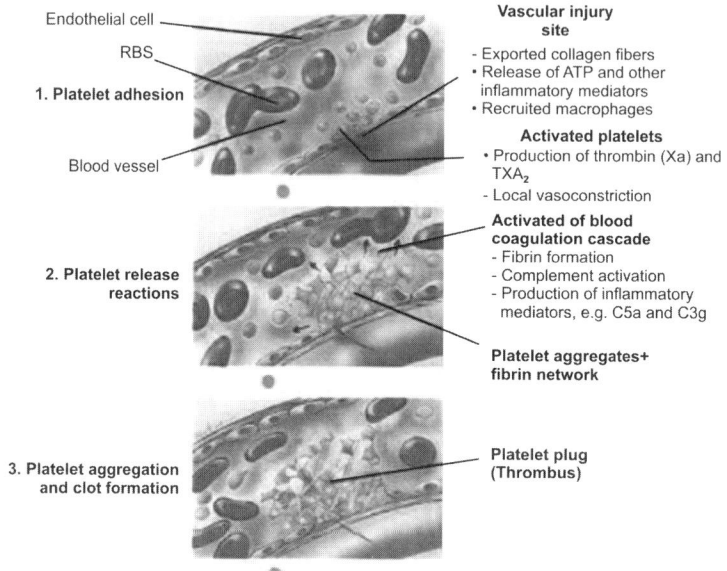

Fig. 9.1 Different steps and components of platelet plug formation in an injured blood vessel

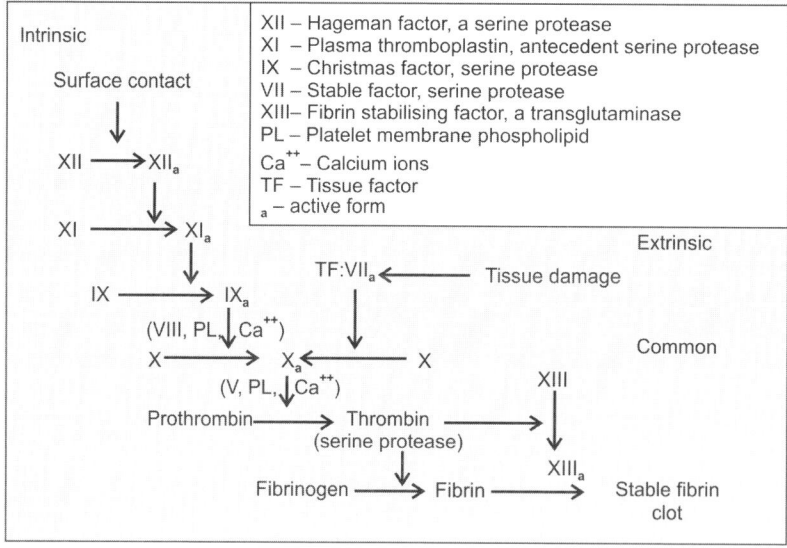

Fig. 9.2 Three pathways that makeup the classical blood coagulation pathway

DENTAL PERSPECTIVE

As a student of Bachelor of Dental Surgery, learning is targeted toward the basic understanding of physiological events of hemostasis and the pathophysiological events associated with coagulation disorders.

Dentists are often required to manage bleeding as part of routine dental procedures or oral surgery and altered hemostasis can lead to complications. Dentist should be aware of impact of bleeding disorders on prognosis and management of their patients. Additionally complex cases of clotting and bleeding disorders requires physician consultation. Comprehensive assessment of data for management includes laboratory tests, diagnosis of the condition, treatment planning with regards to controlling the bleed and careful manipulation of tissues during implementation of treatment protocol for successful management of dental patients with bleeding disorders.

The BT and CT are estimated to evaluate the integrity of the hemostatic mechanism.

Methods for Determination of Bleeding Time

Bleeding time is the time taken from the puncture of the blood vessel to the stoppage of bleeding.

The two methods commonly used for determining the BT are: (1) Duke's method and (2) Ivy's method.

1. Duke's method

The Duke's method is the most commonly used method for estimating the BT.

Principle: The time required for bleeding to stop from the time of giving deep skin puncture is the BT.

Apparatus: Apparatus for sterile puncture (lancet) filter paper and stopwatch.

Procedures

1. Ask the subject to sit comfortably. After explaining the procedure to the subject, the tip of a finger is cleaned with spirit and allowed to dry.
2. Make a puncture deep enough with the help of lancet and ensure free flow of blood without squeezing.
3. Start the stopwatch immediately and note the time of puncture of the finger.
4. Thirty seconds later escaping blood is dried on the edge of a filter paper.
5. The procedure of applying flowing blood on the fresh area of filter paper is continued every 30 seconds till blood ceases to flow.
6. The total number of blood spots on the filter paper is counted and multiplied by 30. This will give the BT in seconds which is converted in minutes. Normal BT by this method is 2–6 minutes.

2. Ivy's method

1. The anterior surface of the forearm is cleaned with spirit.
2. A blood pressure cuff is tied over the subject upper arm and pressure of 40 mmHg is maintained till the end of the experiment.
3. The anterior surface of forearm is cleaned with alcohol and a superficial incision (10 mm long and 1 mm deep) is made with a sterile lancet avoiding visible blood vessels.
4. The blood drops are soaked up every 30 seconds with a piece of filter paper, until the blood no longer stains the paper.

The total number of blood spots on the filter paper is counted and multiply by 30. This will give the BT in seconds which is converted in minutes.

Normal value of bleeding by Ivy method is 3–5 minutes.

Clotting Time (CT)

The time taken from the puncture of the blood vessel to the formation of a fibrin thread is the CT. There are two methods commonly being used for determining the CT: (1) capillary glass tube method and (2) Lee-White method.

A. Capillary glass tube method

This is most commonly used method in practice. These are same steps as described above in Duke's method.

1. The tip of a finger is cleaned with spirit and allowed to dry.
2. Make a puncture deep enough with the help of lancet and ensure free flow of blood without squeezing.
3. When a large drop of blood is collected, the end of the capillary tube is inserted in the drop holding the tube such that its other end will be at a lower level. Blood flows rapidly into the capillary tube.
4. The capillary tube filled with blood is hold in the palm of the hand so as to maintain it at body temperature.
5. Observe for 1 minute and then break off about 1 cu mm of the tube from one end and notice for thread of fibrin if any at the broken ends of the tube. If there is no fibrin thread, the procedure has to be repeated every 30 seconds till a fibrin thread appears. The fibrin thread of about 5 mm length indicates that the blood has clotted.
6. The total time taken from the time of puncture (zero time) till the formation of a fibrin thread is the CT. Normal value of clotting time by this method is 3–8 minutes at 37°C.

B. Lee-White method

1. 2 mL of venous blood is collected under aseptic precaution. The time of vein puncture is noted.
2. The blood is immediately delivered in small tube of 11 mm diameter, and the tube is pre-warmed in a 37°C water bath.
3. Blood clotting is tested by tipping the tube back and forth every 30 seconds.
4. The CT is measured when the blood does not flow out of the test tubes when tilted horizontally.
5. The CT is noted.
6. The normal value is 5–8 minutes.

PRECAUTIONS

1. The finger pricking, incision on forearm or vein puncture should be done under aseptic precaution.
2. The time of finger pricking, incision on forearm or vein puncture should be noted as starting time.

3. The time of stoppage of bleed in BT and formation of fibrin thread in CT estimation should be meticulously noted.
4. Strictly follow the procedure steps and the experiment should be carried out at normal body temperature of 37°C.

Results

1. Bleeding time as per Duke's method
2. Bleeding time as per Ivy's method
3. Clotting time as per capillary tube method
4. Clotting time as per Lee-White method

DENTAL IMPLICATION

The management of patients with bleeding disorders depends on the severity of the condition and the invasiveness of the planned dental procedure. If the procedure has limited invasiveness and the patient has a mild bleeding disorder, only slight or no modification will be required over the standard protocol of management.

In patients with severe bleeding disorders, the goal is to minimize the challenge to the patient by restoring the hemostatic system to acceptable levels and maintaining hemostasis by various local and adjunctive methods. In patients with drug-induced coagulopathies, drugs doses may be modified. The patient's physician should be consulted before invasive treatments are undertaken and drug doses regime are to be followed as per physicians recommendations.

OBJECTIVE STRUCTURED PRACTICAL EXAMINATION (OSPE) QUESTIONS

OSPE I

1. The subject should be explained the procedure and then the tip of a finger is to be cleaned with spirit and allowed to dry. (Yes/No)

2. Making a puncture deep enough with the help of lancet and ensure free flow of blood without squeezing. (Yes/No)

3. Starting the stopwatch immediately and note the time of puncture of the finger. (Yes/No)

4. Thirty seconds later escaping blood is being dried on the edge of a filter paper. (Yes/No)

5. The procedure of applying flowing blood on the fresh area of filter paper is continued every 30 seconds till blood ceases to flow. (Yes/No)

6. The total number of blood spots on the filter paper is counted and multiplied by 30. This will give the BT in seconds which is converted in minutes. Normal BT by this method is 2–6 minutes. (Yes/No)

OSPE II

1. The tip of a finger is cleaned with spirit and allowed to dry.   (Yes/No)

2. A puncture deep enough is made with the help of lancet and ensure   (Yes/No)
   free flow of blood without squeezing.

3. A large drop of blood is collected, the end of the capillary tube is   (Yes/No)
   inserted in the drop holding the tube such that its other end will be
   at a lower level. Blood should flows rapidly into the capillary tube.

4. The capillary tube filled with blood is hold in the palm of the hand   (Yes/No)
   so as to maintain it at body temperature.

5. The procedure of breaking the capillary every 30 seconds till a fibrin   (Yes/No)
   thread appears.

6. The total time taken from the time of puncture (zero time) till the   (Yes/No)
   formation of a fibrin thread is the CT is noted by counting number
   of broken capillary pieces.

VIVA QUESTIONS

1. **Define BT and CT.**

Ans. BT is the time taken from puncture of blood vessel to the stoppage of
bleeding.

   CT is time taken from puncture of blood vessel to formation of a fibrin thread.

2. **How much is the BT as per Duke's method?**

Ans. The normal BT as per Duke's method is 2–6 minutes.

3. **How much is the CT as per capillary glass tube method?**

Ans. The normal CT as per capillary glass tube method is 3–8 minutes at 37°C.

4. **Explain the series of events involved in hemostasis.**

Ans. Three major events which get involved during arrest of bleeding are:

   (i) Constriction of injured blood vessel due to release of 5-HT from the damaged
       platelets
   (ii) Formation of a hemostatic plug of platelets
   (iii) Seal of damaged blood vessel by the blood clot.

5. **Enlist two conditions each in which BT and CT are prolonged.**

Ans. The two conditions in which BT is prolonged are thrombocytopenic purpura and
purpura hemorrhagica.

   The two conditions in which CT is prolonged are hemophilia and vitamin K
deficiency.

6. Discuss the dental management in patients of hemophilia.

Ans. In orthodontic treatment, there are no contraindications in well-motivated patients but careful handling while placement of bands and wires is required.

In operative dentistry, rubber dam should be used to protect tissue against accidental laceration and wedges should be place to protect and retract papilla.

In pulp therapy (which is preferable to extraction), one needs to avoid over instrumentation and overfilling.

In periodontal therapy, there are no contraindications for probing and supra-gingival scaling but deep scaling, curettage and surgery need replacement therapy.

During oral surgery or maxillofacial surgery antifribrinolytic therapy and local hemostatic measure should be judiciously used and is advised not to open lingual tissue in lower molar regions so as to avoid hemorrhage track down an endanger airway.

7. Enlist various dental procedures which have risk of causing bleeding.

Ans. Many dental procedures are associated with bleeding and include dental prophylaxis (teeth cleaning), scaling and root planning (deep teeth cleaning), periodontal (gum) surgery, tooth extractions, dental implant placement and biopsies.

8. What measures are to be advised to the patient to minimize bleeding after a dental procedure?

Ans. As most invasive dental procedures result in bleeding, the patients should be instructed to follow simple procedures like applying firm pressure on the bleeding sites for 10–15 minutes with moist gauze after surgical treatment so that bleeding stops. Patients should be asked to refrain from spitting, rinsing, drinking hot beverages and smoking for at least first 24 hours. The patients should avoid eating hard or sharp foods (pretzels, chips, nuts) for the first 2–3 days.

9. Discuss the appropriate measures to be taken while conducting dental surgery in patients of bleeding disorders.

Ans. The appropriate management for patients with bleeding disorders who require routine invasive dental procedures, restorative procedures or simple surgical procedures should consist of the following:

Step 1: An accurate, comprehensive history of health profile including dental and medication history of the patients should be recorded. Carry a thorough extra and intraoral examination to identify lesions indicative of a bleeding disorder.

Step 2: Consult the supervising physician and obtain additional information about the patient's disorder or bleeding history and pre- and postoperative medication protocol which is to be followed.

Step 3: When performing the invasive procedure one should follow the standard recommended protocol of minimizing tissue trauma. The hemostatic measures in cases of severe bleeding may include the following systemic or local applications: Application of absorbable gelatin sponge containing a thrombin solution; gauze-soaked squares and/or mouth rinses with fibrin or tranexamic acid (TXA); epsilon aminocaproic acid (EACA); vasoconstrictors in local anesthetics and surgical techniques such as suturing.

MULTIPLE CHOICE QUESTIONS

1. The fibrinogen is factor number
   A. I
   B. II
   C. III
   D. IV

2. Prothrombin activator is formed by
   A. Intrinsic pathway
   B. Extrinsic pathway
   C. A and B both
   D. Thrombin

3. The first important event in hemostasis following severe tissue injury is:
   A. Clumping of red blood cells
   B. Vascular spasm
   C. Formation of a platelet hemostatic plug
   D. Formation of thromboplastin

4. The conversion of fibrinogen into fibrin occurs by:
   A. Thrombin
   B. Thrombomodulin
   C. Thromboplastin
   D. Platelets

5. In clotting mechanism via intrinsic and extrinsic pathway, the key reaction is:
   A. Formation of thrombin
   B. Formation of fibrin
   C. Conversion of factor X to its active form
   D. Formation of ATP

6. Intravascular clotting is prevented by circulating:
   A. Heparin
   B. Fibrinolysin
   C. Antithrombin C
   D. All of the above

7. **Fibrinolytic system gets activated by all of the following conditions, except:**
   A. Trypsin inhibitor
   B. Stress and strain
   C. Glucocorticoids
   D. Violent sudden death

8. **Test for clotting is:**
   A. Capillary tube method
   B. Shali's method
   C. Wintrobe's method
   D. Westergren's method

9. **Hemophilia is:**
   A. Autosomal dominant
   B. Autosomal recessive
   C. X-linked recessive
   D. X-linked dominant

10. **In purpura:**
    A. Platelets count may be low
    B. Capillary contractility is defective
    C. CT is normal but BT increases
    D. All of the above

Answers:

1 A	2 C	3 B	4 A	5 C	6 D	7 A	8 A
9 C	10 D						

CLINICAL CASE SCENARIO

Case 1

1. **A 45-year-old male reported for restorative surgery, the patient was on Coumadin therapy. Is it advisable to stop Coumadin therapy of the patient before restorative surgery?**

Ans. Thrombosis may also occur because of a temporary state of rebound hypercoagulability following cessation of anticoagulation therapy. Hence it is advised for physician's review and opinion to be taken before operation and Coumadin therapy should not be stopped.

Case 2

2. **The photograph shows the hemorrhagic complications (a severe hematoma on the anterior floor of the mouth after implant placement in the anterior mandible) after dental implant. Which other complications may be observed in the patient?**

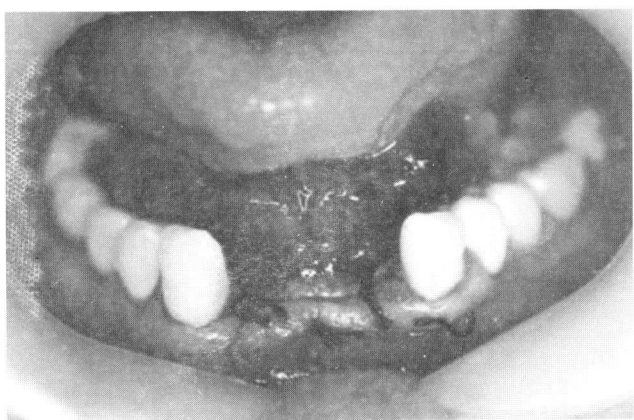

Exhibit 9.1 Hematoma on anterior floor of the mouth

Ans. Due to severe bleeding and the formation of massive hematomas in the floor of the mouth, it can result into an arterial trauma or tearing of the lingual periosteum after dental implant. This occurrence may lead to extensive bleeding into the submandibular space, resulting in a life-threatening acute airway obstruction within the first few hours after surgery. The hemorrhage can easily spread in the loose tissues of the floor of the mouth, the sublingual area and the space between the lingual muscles which may require intubation or an emergency tracheostomy.

Case 3

3. **Identify the pathological cause of bleeding.**

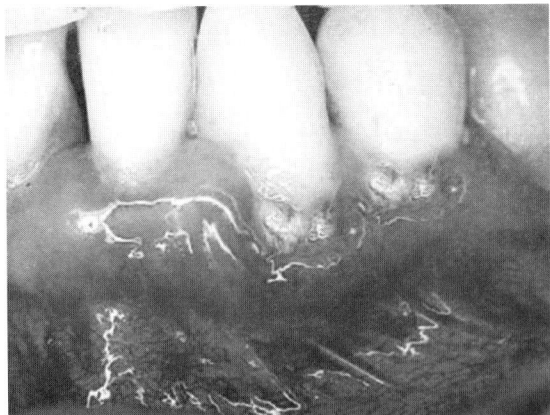

Exhibit 9.2 Bleeding and sore gums

Ans. Bleeding and sore gums as shown in the photograph may be due to gingivitis. This is an early and reversible stage of gum disease as a result of brushing too hard or starting a new flossing routine.

HISTORICAL ASPECT

William Howell and Jay McLean

William Howell was studying procoagulant effects on experimental animals at Johns Hopkins in 1915. Jay McLean joined in laboratory to assist his research work of isolating a thromboplastic material.

Jay McLean found that a phosphatide from the liver, initially procoagulant lost this property and became anticoagulant. McLean informed his mentor Dr Howell that he has discovered antithrombin. McLean named this substance heparphosphatide. Meanwhile, Howell pursued studies on the substance. In 1918, he renamed it heparin.

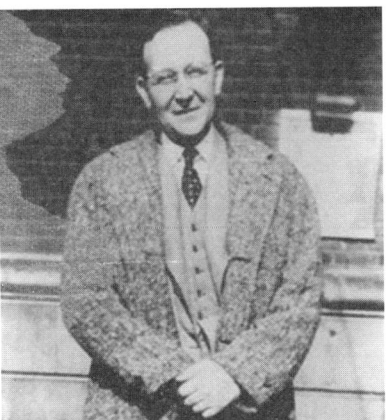

William Howell

Henrik Dam (1895–1976)

In 1929 Henrik Dam, a Danish investigator, found that processed feed was causing hemorrhages in chicks. By 1935, he had isolated prothrombin deficiency as a cause and postulated a sterol vitamin K that would prevent bleeding. The structure of vitamin K was eventually solved by Edward Doisy, and he and Dam received the Nobel Prize in Medicine or Physiology in 1943 for its discovery.

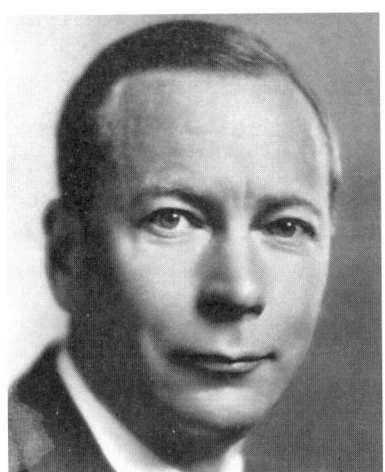

Henrik Dam

RECENT UPDATES

Anticoagulants and antiplatelet drugs are amongst the most commonly used medication. Warfarin and heparin are the most commonly used anticoagulant. The direct thrombin inhibitors a new class of drug (example lepirudin) and small molecular compounds that interfere directly with the enzymatic action of particular coagulation factors (rivaroxaban, dabigatran, apixaban) are under development.

Clinical Examination of Radial Pulse

INTRODUCTION

Arterial pulse is the rhythmic expansion of the arterial wall due to the pressure wave produced by ventricular ejection. The arterial pulse can be felt in the common carotid, brachial, radial, femoral, popliteal and dorsalis pedis arteries. Claudius Galen was perhaps the first physiologist to describe the pulse. The characteristics of pulse are ideally assessed at the radial and carotid arteries. The radial pulse is typically on the radial side of the palmer aspect of the wrist, about 2 cm proximal to the thenar eminence. Radial pulse is best felt when palpated with tips of three middle fingers by mild compression of the vessel against the underlying bone.

DENTAL PERSPECTIVE

As a dentist, you may have to manage the medical emergencies which a patient may land up while being treated in your clinic or on operation table. It may be a cardiac emergency where patient developed myocardial infarction, or anaphylactic reaction due to drug allergy or severe bleeding during procedure as patient had hidden the information that he/she is hypertensive and diabetic, or as incomplete history was revealed by patient regarding his/her cardiac health profile (patient having congenital heart disease or he/she is on anticoagulant therapy). He/she may develop arrhythmias. All dental practitioners should be able to immediately provide basic first aid care such as ensuring adequate airway, breathing and circulation. One should immediately record the pulse, blood pressure and respiratory rate and shift the patient to the medical casualty.

Aim: To examine the radial pulse in a human subject.

Method:
1. Ask the subject to sit comfortably on examination stool.
2. Ask the subject to keep his/her forearm semipronated and the wrist slightly flexed.
3. Palpate the radial pulse using his/her index, middle and ring finger by placing the fingers along the radial side of the palmer aspect of the wrist, about 2 cm proximal to the thenar eminence.

Take note of the following features of the pulse:

Rate: Examine the radial pulse by palpating radial artery and count the pulse of the subject for 1 minute. Take three readings, and take the mean value. The normal pulse rate ranges between 60 and 100/min in an adult. It is an accurate indication of the heart rate in a normal person. Tachycardia is defined as a pulse rate more than 100/min and bradycardia as a rate less than 60/min.

Rhythm: Normally, the pulse has a regular rhythm. Assess the interval between consecutive pulses. Confirm whether the rhythm is regular or irregular. In disease, the rhythm may be regularly irregular or irregularly irregular.

The heart rate increases during inspiration and slows during expiration. It is called respiratory sinus arrhythmia and it is most obvious in children, young adults and athletes.

Volume or amplitude: Volume is the term used to indicate the impulse up thrust imparted to a finger on palpating the pulse. Volume is ascessed by the perception of expansion of the arterial wall. The pulse is weak or thready in heart failure, circulatory shock and aortic stenosis. The pulse is high volume and strong in pregnancy, thyrotoxicosis, aortic regurgitation, hyperthermia or after heavy exercise.

Character: It refers to an impression of the pulse waveform derived during palpation. Again, like volume, it needs to be examined at one of the large arteries. Alterations in the rate, rhythm and volume alter the normal character of the arterial pulse. Altered character of the pulse is seen in anacrotic pulse, dicrotic pulse, pulsus paradoxus, pulsus alternans, water-hammer pulse or collapsing pulse, pulsus bisiferens, etc.

Condition of the arterial wall: Obliterate the blood flow in the radial artery by pressing your index finger against bony prominence. Empty the radial artery peripherally using the ring finger. You have to feel for the condition of the vessel wall by rolling the segment of the radial artery on the underlying bone using your middle finger.

Compare the radial pulse on both sides.

Examine other peripheral pulses, namely the carotid, brachial, femoral, popliteal, and dorsalis pedis arteries.

Radiofemoral delay: Examine for any delay between radial and femoral pulses.

Results

1. Pulse rate is _____/minute
2. Rhythm: Regular/irregular
3. Volume: Adequate/high/low
4. Condition of the vessel wall: Soft/hard rigid
5. Radiofemoral delay, if any: Yes/No
6. Other peripheral artery: _____

DENTAL IMPLICATION

Literature states that major medical emergencies occur during root canal therapy or extraction procedures. Many dental procedures require the patient to undergo general anesthesia. The patients who are high-risk for anaphylactic reactions or in critical health need to be monitored. Monitoring a patient's vitals of pulse and blood pressure during the procedures or operations is crucial to ensure the patient's safety. Monitoring of vitals especially pulse and blood pressure helps the dental clinician to identify acute medical emergencies which could require immediate attention.

OBJECTIVE STRUCTURED PRACTICAL EXAMINATION (OSPE) QUESTIONS

1. **Examine the pulse of the individual sitting for clinical examination.**
   - Ensures palm is warm before touching the patient. (Yes/No)
   - Palpate the radial artery with the tips of the index and middle fingers. (Yes/No)
   - Does not press too hard for fear of obliterating the pulse. (Yes/No)
   - Counts the pulse for a minute. (Yes/No)

Identify the arterial pulse wave and interpret the same.

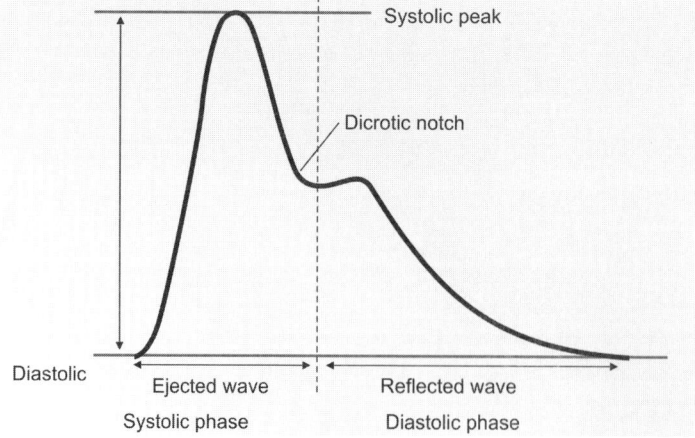

Fig. 10.1 Diagrammatic representation of a radial arterial pulse wave

It is the radial arterial pulse wave and forms a contour wave which is generated by the heart when it contracts, and it travels along the arterial walls of the arterial tree. Pulse waveform has two components: Forward moving wave and a reflected wave. The forward wave is generated when the ventricles contracts during systole. The reflected wave appears in the diastolic phase, after the closure of the aorta valves. Dicrotic notch is the sudden drop in pressure after systolic contraction.

VIVA QUESTIONS

1. **What are the various reasons for irregular rhythm of pulse?**

Ans. An irregular pulse may be due to sinus arrhythmia, premature beats, ectopic beats, atrial fibrillation, paroxysmal atrial tachycardia, atrial flutter, partial heart block, etc.

2. **Enlist a few conditions in which hyperkinetic pulse are seen.**

Ans. Hyperkinetic pulse is seen in fever, anemia, thyrotoxicosis, hyperkinetic heart syndrome, A-V fistula, Paget's disease, beriberi, etc.

3. **Name the conditions in which an unequal pulse is seen between upper and lower extremities.**

Ans. The unequal pulse is seen between upper and lower extremities in coarctation of aorta, aortitis, block at bifurcation of aorta, dissection of aorta, iatrogenic trauma and arteriosclerotic obstruction.

4. **Locate the position for palpation of femoral artery and dorsalis pedis artery.**

Ans. Femoral pulse is located in the inner thigh at the mid-inguinal point, halfway between the pubic symphysis and the anterior superior iliac spine (femoral artery). The dorsalis pedis pulse is located on top of the foot, immediately lateral to the extensor of hallucis longus.

5. **Which precautions are to be taken while palpating carotid artery?**

Ans. The carotid artery is to be palpated gently while the patient is sitting or lying down. The two carotid arteries should not be palpated at the same time. This may limit the flow of blood to the head, possibly leading to fainting or brain ischemia. The student should be aware that stimulating its baroreceptors with low palpitation can provoke severe bradycardia or even stop the heart in nervous subjects.

MULTIPLE CHOICE QUESTIONS

1. **Hypokinetic pulse is seen in:**
   A. Congestive cardiac failure
   B. A-V fistula
   C. Paget's disease
   D. Thyrotoxicosis

2. **Force of pulse is known as compressibility of pulse and it is a rough measure of:**
   A. Systolic blood pressure
   B. Diastolic pressure
   C. Pulse pressure
   D. Mean blood pressure

3. **A discrepant or unequal pulse between left and right radial artery is observed in:**
   A. Anomalous or aberrant course of artery
   B. Coarctation of aorta
   C. Aortitis
   D. Dissecting aneurysm
   E. All of the above

4. **A thick radial artery which is palpable up to _____ is suggestive of arteriosclerosis.**
   A. 7.5–10 cm up the forearm
   B. 1.5–2 cm up the forearm
   C. 3–4 cm
   D. None of the above

5. **Radiofemoral delay is seen in:**
   A. Coarctation of aorta
   B. Myocardial infarction
   C. Angina
   D. Asthma

Answers:

1 A	2 A	3 D	4 A	5 A

HISTORICAL ASPECT

Claudius Galen

Claudius Galen was a Greek physician born in 131 AD and died in 201 AD. He was a gifted intellect who studied at the famous medical school in Alexandria in Egypt. Galen was greatly influenced by the working methods of Hippocrates. He placed great importance on clinical observation through careful examination of patients and the recording of their symptoms. Galen advocated that

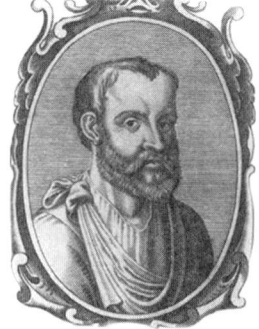

Claudius Galen

pulse should be monitored meticulously and is important to detect it for abnormalities and it should be used as a tool to diagnose disease and suggest possible treatments.

RECENT UPDATES

The remote patient monitoring (RPM) enables monitoring of patients outside of conventional clinical settings may be office, home, leisure places etc., and this increases access to care and reduces healthcare delivery costs. Wireless body area network (WBAN) integrates intelligent, miniaturized, low-power sensor nodes within, around or over a human body to monitor body functions.

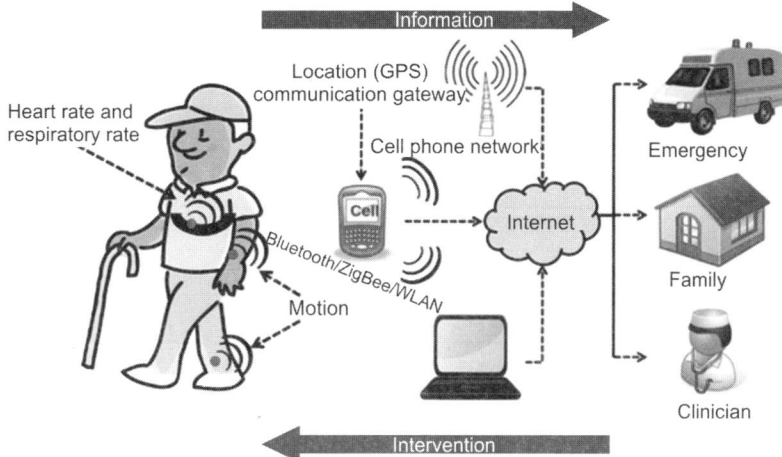

Exhibit 10.1 Remote patient monitoring and patient care

Physiological data such as blood pressure, pulse, heart rate and ECG can be collected by sensors on peripheral devices. This helps in timely assistance in cases of casualty and emergencies and ensures positive patient outcomes. The newer applications also provide education, test and medication reminder alerts, and a means of communication between the patient and the provider. This is revolutionizing the future of healthcare technology.

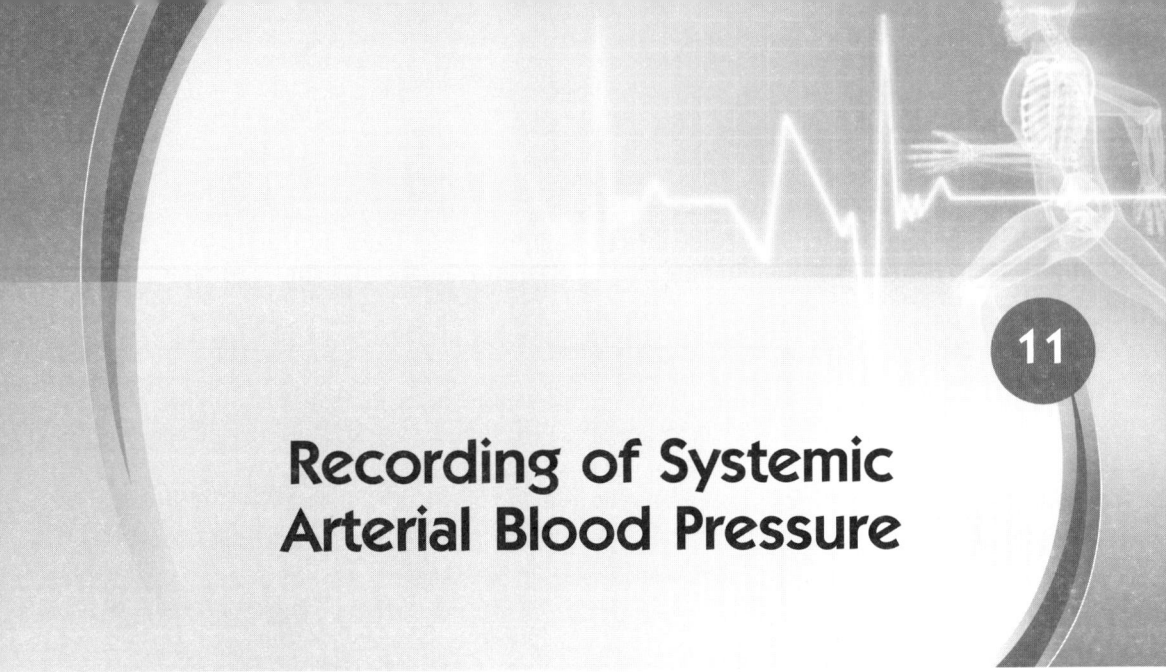

Recording of Systemic Arterial Blood Pressure

11

Learning Objectives

After learning the practicals, the student should be able to:

1. Define blood pressure. Explain the terms systolic, diastolic, mean blood pressure and pulse pressure.
2. List factors that influence blood pressure.
3. Demonstrate how to take blood pressure by palpatory and auscultatory methods.
4. Explain the precautions to be taken while recording the blood pressure.
5. Explain the short-term and long-term regulatory mechanism of blood pressure.
6. Explain regarding the importance of recording blood pressure before and after dental surgery.
7. Discuss the lifestyle modification activities to control blood pressure.

INTRODUCTION

Arterial blood pressure is the lateral pressure exerted on arterial wall by the column of blood while flowing through it.

The first time determination of arterial blood pressure was done by Rev Stephen Hales in the year 1733 in mare as experimental animal by inserting a brass cannula into the central end of femoral artery. He tied the cannula to a long glass which was having height of 3 meters. Rev Stephen Hales observed the oscillation and rise of blood column.

Riva Rocci invented the sphygmomanometer in the year 1886. Sphygmomanometer was thereafter used to record blood pressure in human beings.

DEFINITIONS

Systolic blood pressure: It is the maximum pressure excreted during systole. The normal value is 120 mmHg (100–120 mmHg).

Diastolic blood pressure: It is the minimum pressure exerted during the diastole. The normal value is 80 mmHg.

Mean Arterial blood pressure: It is the average pressure exerted during the cardiac cycle. Mean blood pressure (MBP) is expressed as diastolic blood pressure +1/3rd of pulse pressure. The average mean blood pressure is 96 mmHg and ranges between 95 mmHg and 100 mmHg.

Pulse Pressure: The difference between the diastolic and systolic blood pressure is the pulse pressure. Normal range of pulse pressure averages around 40 mmHg.

DENTAL PERSPECTIVE

World Health Organization attributes hypertension or high blood pressure as the leading cause of cardiovascular mortality. An elevated arterial pressure is probably the most important public health problem in developed countries. It is a professional responsibility of a dental clinician to carefully examine vitals including blood pressure and informs the patient of their hypertensive state and to offer medical advice including appropriate referrals. There are no recognized oral manifestations of hypertension but antihypertensive drugs can often cause side-effects such as xerostomia, gingival overgrowth, erythema multiform, lichenoid drug reactions, taste sense alteration and parasthesia.

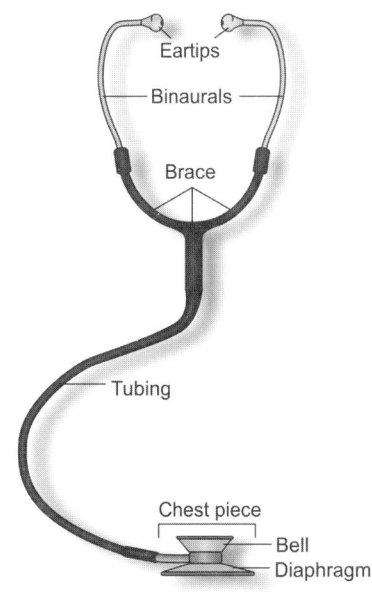

DETERMINATION OF BLOOD PRESSURE

Apparatus

Stethoscope: The stethoscope is used to auscultate the Korotkoff sound. The parts of stethoscope includes:

a. Chest piece: It has the bell and diaphragm as two end pieces.

b. Ear frame: It has two curved metallic tubes (binaurals) approximated together to the y-shaped spring (braces). The y-shaped connector connects the metal tube to the chest piece. The plastic knobs are attached to the curved metallic tube at their open end and it facilitates comfortable feeling in the ear.

Fig. 11.1 Stethoscope

Sphygmomanometer

The sphygmomanometer is the instrument used for recording arterial blood pressure in humans. The sphygmomanometer consists of the following parts:

a. **Mercury manometer:** One arm of the manometer is for the reservoir for mercury and contains enough mercury to be driven up in the other limb which is the graduated glass tube.

b. **Manometer graduated glass tube:** It is graduated in mm from 0 to 300 mmHg, each division representing 2 mm. A stopcock between the two limbs when closed prevents the mercury from entering the glass tube. The one-way valve fitted at the top of the mercury well prevents spilling of mercury when the lid is closed.

c. **Cuff:** It consists of an inflatable rubber bag having length of 24 cm and width of 12 cm and is fitted with two rubber tubes, one connecting it to the mercury reservoir and the other to a long strip of inelastic cloth. The cloth covering keeps the rubber bag in position around the arm when arterial blood pressure is being measured. As a general rule, the width of the bag is 20% more than the arm diameter.

d. **Hand bulb (rubber bulb):** The oval-shaped rubber bulb has a one-way valve at its free end, and a leak-valve with a knurled screw at the other end where the rubber tube leading to the cuff is attached. The cuff can be inflated by turning the leak valve screw clockwise and deflation of the bag is achieved by turning this screw anticlockwise.

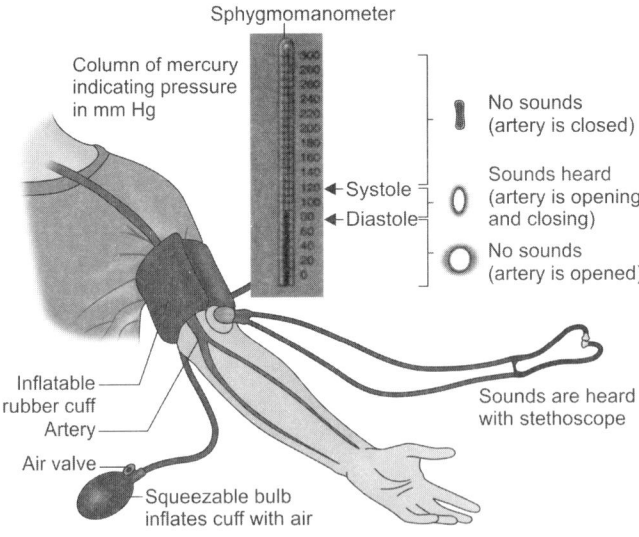

Fig. 11.2 Sphygmomanometer

Aneroid manometer: The calibrated dial replaces the mercury manometer in aneroid manometer.

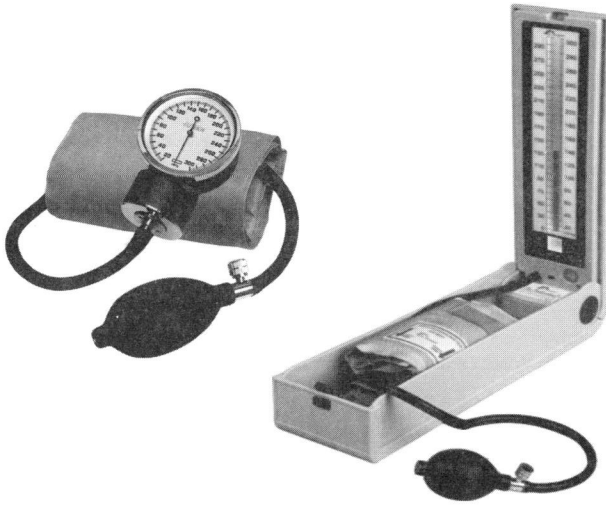

Fig. 11.3 Aneroid and mercurial sphygmomanometer

Procedures

It can be determined by the direct and indirect methods.

- The direct methods (cannulation) are:
  a. Optical manometer
  b. Electrical transducer

Nowadays the direct methods are used during research experimentation in animals.

- The indirect methods are:
  a. Oscillatory method
  b. Palpatory method
  c. Auscultatory method

Oscillatory Method

The vibration produced by passing of blood through narrow channels (turbulent flow) produces oscillation indicating the pressure in the arteries. This method is no longer used.

Palpatory Method

The systolic pressure is determined by feeling the pulsation of radial artery after inflating or deflating the cuff over the upper arm.

Steps for measuring blood pressure using palpatory method

1. Make the subject lie comfortably on the examination couch or subject is asked to sit comfortably on a chair.

2. Wrap the cuff along the exposed arm of the subject and ensure that the midpoint of the cuff overlies the brachial artery and the lower edge of the cuff is around 1 inch above the cubital fossa at the heart level.
3. Palpate the radial artery pulsation at the wrist and inflate the cuff until the arm pressure within it overcomes the arterial pressure, thereby obliterating the lumen of the artery and this is confirmed by the disappearance of the radial artery pulsation.
4. The cuff pressure should be raised by 30 mmHg. Now deflate the cuff at the rate of 2–3 mmHg/s while continue feeling radial artery pulsation.
5. Watch over the reading on the manometer scale when radial artery pulsation disappears. This gives the systolic blood pressure by the palpatory method.

Advantage of the palpatory method: The fallacy of auscultatory method in missing the auscultatory gap is avoided in palpatory method.

Disadvantages of the palpatory method
1. The diastolic pressure cannot be measured by this method.
2. The systolic blood pressure measured is lower than the actual systolic blood pressure by 4–6 mmHg. When the cuff pressure just balances the brachial artery pressure, only a small amount of blood flow through the artery which may not be sufficient enough to generate a pulse wave.

Auscultatory Method

Preparation of the subject
1. **Rapport with the subject:** Ensure that you introduce yourself to the patient, explain the procedure, answer any question he may have and ask for his consent. Make sure he is sitting comfortably with his arm rested at the heart level.
2. **Positioning** (level): While taking the reading, the eye should be at the level of the mercury column, to avoid parallax errors while subjects arm should be held at heart level.
3. **Placement:** Ensure correct placement of the cuff. Wrap the cuff around the patient's upper arm ensuring the lower edge of the cuff is placed 1 inch above the antecubital fossa. The bladder of the cuff should be centered over brachial artery (palpate medial to biceps tendon). Fasten the cuff evenly and snugly.
4. **Performance:**
   a. The brachial artery determines a rough value for the systolic blood pressure. This can be done by palpating the brachial or radial pulse and inflating the cuff until the pulse can no longer be felt. The reading at this point should be noted and the cuff deflated.
   b. Place the diaphragm of your stethoscope over the brachial artery and re-inflate the cuff to 20–30 mmHg higher than the estimated value taken before. Then deflate the cuff at 2–3 mmHg per second until the light taping sound is heard. Continue to lower the pressure in the cuff and appreciate the change in the quality and intensity of the sounds heard through the stethoscope. These are called Korotkoff's sounds after the Russian scientist Korotkoff who described these sounds in 1905. He differentiated five phases of these sounds (see figure).

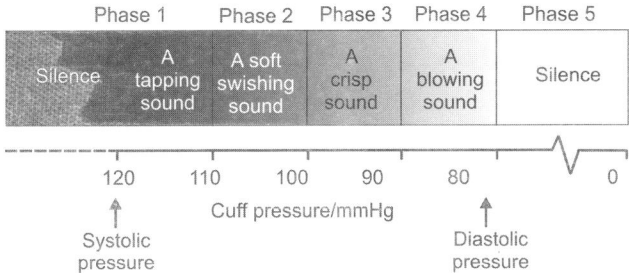

Phase 1	Phase 2	Phase 3	Phase 4	Phase 5
Silence	A tapping sound	A soft swishing sound	A crisp sound	A blowing sound	Silence

120   110   100   90   80   0

Cuff pressure/mmHg

↑ Systolic pressure

↑ Diastolic pressure

Table 11.1 Phase by characterstics of sound produced while recording arterial blood pressure

- **Phase 1 (K1):** Clear tapping sounds representing systolic pressure.
- **Phase 2 (K2):** Onset of swishing sound or murmur
- **Phase 3 (K3):** Loud slapping crisp sound
- **Phase 4 (K4):** A blowing sound getting muffled representing diastolic pressure
- **Phase 5 (K5):** Tones cease

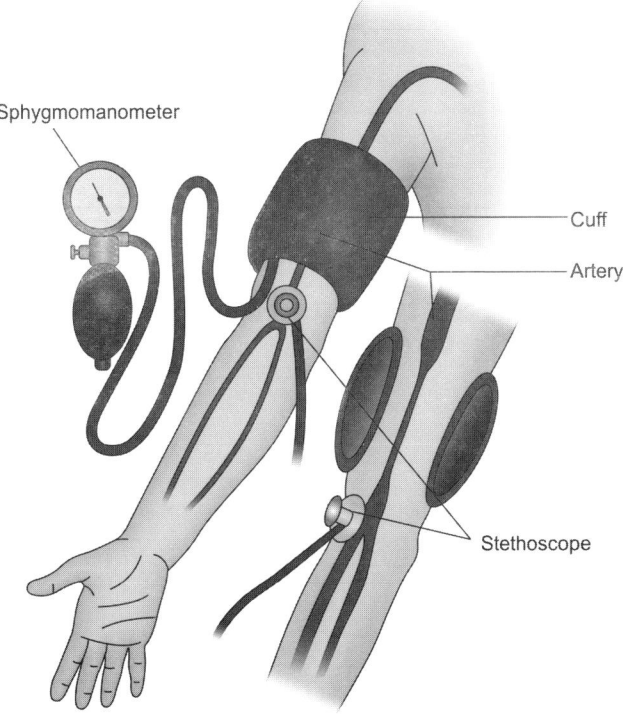

Sphygmomanometer

Cuff

Artery

Stethoscope

Fig. 11.4 Sketch diagram representing the cuff and stethoscope positioning while recording blood pressure

Precaution

- The subject should be made to relax for 5–10 minutes before blood pressure is recorded.
- Level: While taking the reading, the eye should be at the level of the mercury column, in order to avoid parallax errors the subjects arm should be held at heart level.
- Wrap the cuff around the patient's upper arm ensuring the lower edge of the cuff is placed 1 inch above the antecubital fossa. The bladder of the cuff should be centered over brachial artery (palpate medial to biceps tendon).
- The cuff should not be tied too loose or too tight.
- The cuff pressure should be reduced to zero between the trials. Otherwise, inflated cuff will produce reflex spasm of the artery and false reading.
- The mercury column should be deflated slowly at the rate of 2–3 mm/sec, otherwise they will be underestimated systolic blood pressure value.

Results

1. **Normal values:** Normally, in adults the systolic pressure ranges between 100 mmHg and 140 mmHg, and the diastolic pressure between 60 mmHg and 90 mmHg.

2. Take the average of three readings and note the result.

3. Name of the subject: _____   Age: _____

4. Blood pressure recording: _____

5. Systolic blood pressure: _____

6. Diastolic blood pressure: _____

OBJECTIVE STRUCTURED CLINICAL EXAMINATION (OSCE) QUESTIONS

Record the Blood Pressure of the Subject

The following steps should be followed to record the blood pressure.

1. Ensure that you have the following necessary equipment: A sphygmo-   (Yes/No)
   manometer, a stethoscope, hand cleansing gel (equipment for
   measuring blood pressure).

2. Rapport with the subject: Ensure that you introduce yourself to the   (Yes/No)
   patient. Explain the procedure answering any question they may
   have and ask for their consent. Make sure they are sitting comfortably
   with their arm rested.

3. Positioning (*level*): Devices and columns at eye level, patient's arm   (Yes/No)
   held at heart level.

4. Placement: Ensure correct placement of the cuff. Wrap the cuff around   (Yes/No)
   the patient's upper arm ensuring the lower edge of the cuff is placed
   1 inch above the ante-cubital fossa. The bladder of the cuff should be
   centered over brachial artery (palpate medial to biceps tendon). Fasten
   the cuff evenly and snugly.

5. Performance:

a. The brachial artery determines a rough value for the systolic blood   (Yes/No)
pressure. This can be done by palpating the brachial or radial pulse
and inflating the cuff until the pulse can no longer be felt. The
reading at this point should be noted and the cuff deflated.

b. Place the diaphragm of your stethoscope over the brachial artery   (Yes/No)
and reinflate the cuff to 20–30 mmHg higher than the estimated
value taken before. Then deflate the cuff at 2–3 mmHg per
second until you hear the first Korotkoff sound—this is the
systolic blood pressure.

c. Continue to deflate the cuff until the sounds disappear. This is   (Yes/No)
the diastolic blood pressure. Record the true blood pressure.

VIVA QUESTIONS

1. **Define blood pressure, systolic blood pressure, diastolic blood pressure, mean blood pressure and pulse pressure.**

Ans. • **Blood pressure** is the lateral pressure exerted on the wall of the arterial vessels by the contained blood.

• **Systolic blood pressure** is the maximum pressure exerted during the systole. The normal value is 120 mmHg (100–120 mmHg).

• **Diastolic blood pressure** is the minimum pressure exerted during the diastole. The normal value is 80 mmHg (60–80 mmHg)

• **Pulse pressure:** The difference between systolic and diastolic blood pressure is called the pulse pressure. It averages around 40 mmHg.

• **Mean blood pressure** is the average of systolic and diastolic blood pressure, for example, 120 + 80/2 = 100 mmHg. But mean pressure can be more accurately determined by the following equation:

Mean pressure = Diastolic blood pressure + 1/3rd of pulse pressure.

It averages between 95 mmHg and 100 mmHg.

2. **What is peripheral resistance? What are the factors affecting it?**

Ans. It is the fractional resistance offered by the circulatory system to the flow of blood. The factors affecting peripheral resistance are:

a. Viscosity of the blood

b. Size of the lumen of the blood vessels

c. Velocity of blood flow.

3. **What is orthostatic hypotension? What are its causes?**

Ans. It is postural hypotension in which patients on sudden standing from sitting or lying down position experience dizziness, dimension of vision, decreased systemic blood pressure and loss of consciousness.

The causes are:

a. Autonomic insufficiency secondary to lower basal norepinephrine level and in patients of diabetes mellitus and syphilis.

b. Those on sympatholytic drugs.

c. Primary hyperaldosteronism (these patients having abnormal baroreceptor reflex).

4. What is the effect of exercise on blood pressure?

Ans. The systolic blood pressure after exercise rises because of increased cardiac output, as a result of increased myocardial contractibility and sympathetic stimulation. Depending on the degree of exercise the diastolic blood pressure is affected. Diastolic blood pressure increases in mild exercise due to vasoconstriction and does not change or even may decrease in moderate exercise but may fall in intense exercise due to increases body temperature and vasodilatation because of accumulation of metabolites.

5. Explain the important short-term and intermediate mechanism of regulation of blood pressure.

Ans. These mechanisms are:

A. **Neural (short-term regulation) mechanism:** There are three different neural mechanisms.

1. *Baroreceptor reflex* (Marey's reflex): These receptors are located in the carotid sinus and aortic arch which respond to the stretch. They act by decreasing or increasing the sympathetic and vagal tone through vasomotor center and cardioinhibitory center, thus either BP is increased or decreased.

2. *Chemoreceptor reflex:* These receptors responsive to hypoxia, hypercapnia and acidosis are present in the carotid body and aortic body. They act through the respiratory center and come into action once the BP dips below 60 mmHg. Low P (O_2) and/or high P (CO_2) levels in the arterial blood cause reflex increases in respiratory rate and mean arterial pressure.

3. *Cushing's reflex:* Also known as last ditch effort. This reflex comes into play when BP is below 40 mmHg and is due to ischemia of brain or increased intracranial pressure.

B. **Renal mechanism (long-term regulation):** Renin-angiotensin system: Renin is a glycoprotein produced by the juxtaglomerular cells of the kidney in an inactive form called prorenin. Whenever there is a fall in BP, the blood supply to kidney is reduced which stimulates the release of renin in circulation. Renin is converted to active renin by action of kallikreins.

The renin acts on angiotensin to form angiotensin I.

This angiotensin I is converted to angiotensin II and then III by angiotensin-converting enzyme and angiotensinase.

The angiotensin II and III increase the peripheral resistance, blood volume, cardiac output and thus blood pressure by vasoconstriction, aldosterone secretion which causes water and Na^+ reabsorption from tubules, ADH secretion and stimulation of thirst center.

6. Define hypertension.

Ans. Hypertension is the persistent rise in systolic arterial pressure above 140–160 mmHg and diastolic arterial pressure above 90 mm Hg.

7. Define hypotension. What are its causes?

Ans. A persistent fall in basal diastolic blood pressure below 80 mmHg. The causes of hypotension are:

Table 11.2 Cardiac and vascular origins of arterial hypotension

8. What are the oral dental diseases associated with hypertension?

Ans. There are no recognized oral manifestations of hypertension but antihypertensive drugs can often cause side-effects such as xerostomia, gingival overgrowth, erythema multiform, lichenoid drug reactions, taste sense alteration and parasthesia.

9. What is the effect of posture on blood pressure?

Ans. In erect posture there is peripheral pooling of the blood in the dependent parts decreasing venous return to heart and thereby decreases cardiac output and the blood pressure. This increases the discharge of baroreceptor by sympathetic stimulation and increase arterial resistance which increases systolic and diastolic pressure.

In lying down position, the systolic and diastolic blood pressure decreases. The systolic and diastolic blood pressure remains at physiological level (normal) in sitting position.

10. What are the factors affecting blood pressure?

Ans. The factors affecting blood pressure are:

1. **Age:** Blood pressure increases with age.

Newborn: The systolic blood pressure averages around 40 mmHg.

Children: Systolic blood pressure is 90–110 mmHg and diastolic blood pressure is between 50 mmHg and 80 mmHg.

Adult: Systolic blood pressure is between 100 mmHg and 140 mmHg and diastolic blood pressure is between 60 mmHg and 90 mmHg.

2. **Sex:** Blood pressure in females is less than males in the same age group prior to menopause.

3. **Diet:** Blood pressure increases after food intake as it increases metabolic rate.

4. **Environmental temperature:** Blood pressure increases during winter when environmental temperature is low due to vasoconstriction. It decreases during summer when environmental temperature is high due to vasodilatation.

5. **Emotional status:** Anxiety and anger raises the blood pressure due to increase in sympathetic discharges.

6. **Sleep and rest:** Sleep and rest condition decreases the blood pressures.

7. **Exercise:** It causes rise in systolic blood pressure and fall in diastolic blood pressure. The fall in diastolic blood pressure is due to accumulation of metabolites.

11. **What lifestyle modification will you advice to a hypertensive patient?**

Ans. These steps include maintaining a healthy weight; being physically active; following a healthy eating plan that emphasizes fruits, vegetables and low fat dairy foods; choosing and preparing foods with less salt and sodium; and if you drink alcoholic beverages, drinking in moderation is advised.

MULTIPLE CHOICE QUESTIONS

1. The sphygmomanometer was invented in 1886 by:
   A. Riva Rocci
   B. Stephen Hales
   C. Kortokoff
   D. Alexander Fleming

2. Direct method of recording blood pressure is:
   A. Palpatory method
   B. By electrical transducer
   C. Oscillatory method
   D. Auscultatory method

3. The following smooth muscle relaxant reduces blood pressure:
   A. Hydralazine
   B. Phenyl-epinephrine
   C. Adrenaline
   D. Noradrenaline

4. **Marey's law states that:**
   A. Pulse rate is inversely proportional to respiratory rate
   B. BMR is inversely proportional to heart rate
   C. Respiratory rate is inversely proportional to heart rate
   D. Blood pressure is inversely proportional to heart rate

5. **Mean blood pressure is:**
   A. Systolic BP + 1/3rd of diastolic blood pressure
   B. Diastolic BP + 1/3rd of pulse pressure
   C. Pulse pressure + 1/3rd of systolic blood pressure
   D. Diastolic blood pressure – systolic blood pressure

6. **In sudden change of posture from standing to lying down position:**
   A. Systolic blood pressure falls
   B. Diastolic blood pressure increases
   C. Peripheral pooling of blood and increase in heart rate and venous return
   D. All of the above

7. **Which of the following mechanisms regulate the fall in blood pressure?**
   A. Baroreceptor reflex
   B. Capillary fluid shift mechanism
   C. Chemoreceptor reflex
   D. All of the above

8. **Lichen planus infection in oral cavity is commonly seen in patent administering:**
   A. Aspirin for fever
   B. Penicillin
   C. Captopril as anti-hypertensive
   D. Pseudoephedrine

9. **Gingival hypertrophy is seen in patient administering:**
   A. Chlormphenicol
   B. Captopril as anti-hypertensive
   C. Phenytoin sodium
   D. Diazepam

10. **Administering adrenaline as local anesthetic while performing dental procedure should be used cautiously in patient of:**
    A. Hypertension
    B. Sickle cell anemia
    C. Protein energy malnutrition
    D. Respiratory tract infection

11. **The most common cause of hypotension is:**
    A. Acute loss of blood or fluid
    B. Pheochromocytoma
    C. Eclampsia
    D. Renal artery stenosis

12. **The most effective nervous mechanism which returns the BP back to normal is:**
    A. Baroreceptor reflex
    B. Chemoreceptor reflex
    C. Renin angiotensin system
    D. Capillary fluid shift mechanism

13. **Match the following**

Cause	Mechanism
A. Polycythemia	1. Excess aldosterone secretion leading to salt and water retention
B. Pheochromocytoma	2. Mineralocorticoid activity of estrogen and progesterone.
C. Conn's disease	3. Tumor of adrenal medulla leading to excess secretion of adrenaline and noradrenaline.
D. Long-term oral contraceptive use	4. Increased viscosity of blood leading to higher peripheral resistance.

Answers:

1 A	2 B	3 A	4 D	5 B	6 C	7 D	8 C
9 B	10 A	11 A	12 A	13 A-4	B-3	C-1	D-2

APPLIED CLINICAL PHYSIOLOGY IN DENTAL PRACTICE

High Blood Pressure: Effects on Oral Health

Medications that are used to treat hypertension can have effects on the oral environment. Some may cause patients to experience dry mouth, also known as xerostomia. Xerostomia may result in gingivitis, periodontal disease or due to erosion, loss of tooth structure. If left untreated, xerostomia will lower the pH within the oral cavity which increases the development of plaque and therefore dental caries. An altered sense of taste (dysgeusia) is another effect of hypertension medications may have on the oral cavity as well as some others may make patients more likely to faint when raised in a dental chair too quickly which is a reaction known as orthostatic hypotension. Gingival overgrowth (gingival hyperplasia) is another possible side-effect of medications used to treat high blood pressure, for example, calcium channel blockers can often have this effect. Some patients will have to undergo gingival surgery to remove some of the gingiva, but quite often it will just grow back.

CLINICAL CASE SCENARIO

1. A male patient aged 42 years came to dental clinic with complaints of difficulty in eating and reported to be on calcium channel blocker for his treatment for hypertension. Identify the dental pathology from the photograph and explain the causes for the disease condition.

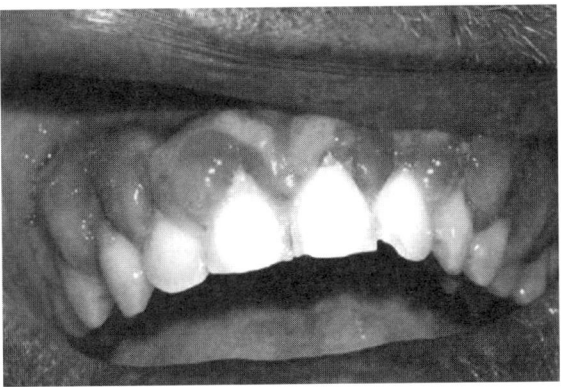

Exhibit 11.1 Gingival enlargement

Ans. The patient is having gingival enlargements due to antihypertensive therapy for his hypertension. Gingival enlargement is also one of the most common clinical findings in patients with hypertension taking antihypertensive medication especially calcium channel blockers. It appears clinically as firm nodules of gingival overgrowth seen on either lingual or palatal aspects or buccal or facial aspects of the marginal gingiva. It may involve the entire crown, thereby causes difficulty in eating. Amlodipine and nifedipine are other drugs which may cause gingival enlargement.

2. What is drug induced gingival overgrowth (DIGO)? How can gingival overgrowth be reduced?

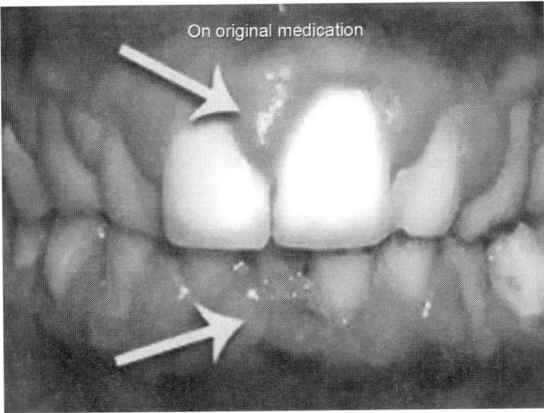

On original medication

Exhibit 11.1 Gingival overgrowth

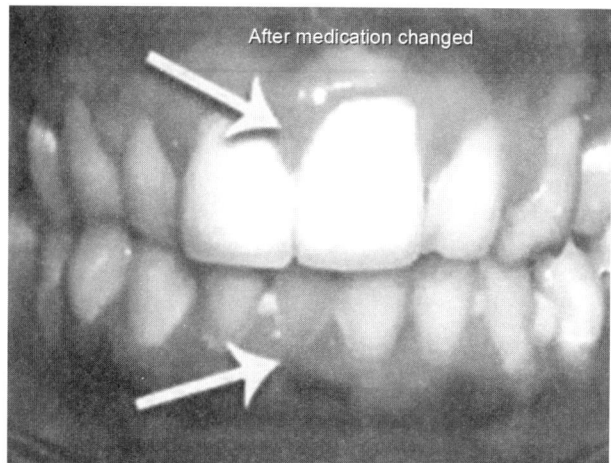

Exhibit 11.3 Regression of gingival hyperplasia

Ans. The drugs that cause DIGO are phenytoin, cyclosporine and calcium channel blockers including nifedipine, diltiazem and amlodipine. Changing of drug has found usually causes regression of gingival hyperplasia provided the oral hygiene is excellent.

3. **A 49-year-old healthy looking male reported for tooth extraction. The blood pressure and vitals were in normal physiological limits. He was administered epinephrine as anesthesia. He developed headache and reported of chest pain while the procedure was being completed. Later, while on dental chair as he felt uneasy he reported that he was on antihypertensive therapy. What can be the reason for his complaints?**

Ans. Epinephrine is a common additive in local anesthetic products. Use of epinephrine in some patients with high blood pressure may result in cardiovascular changes including the rapid rise in blood pressure, angina, heart attack and arrhythmias and these drugs should be used with caution. Hence the dental surgeon should take detail clinical history and record blood pressure before starting any operative procedure.

4. **What kind of anesthesia should be administered in patient who is on Anti-hypertensive drugs?**

Ans. The total dosage of epinephrine should be limited to 0.04 mg in cardiac risk patients. The use of one to two 1.8 mL cartridges of local anesthetic containing a vasoconstrictor is of a little clinical significance for most patients with hypertension on antihypertensive therapy (beta-adrenergic drugs, such as propranolol or cardioselective beta-blockers like lopressor or tenormin), and this dose will have minimal physiologic effect and provides prolonged anesthesia. The benefits of maintaining adequate anesthesia for the duration of the procedure far outweighs the risks.

HISTORICAL ASPECT

Stephen Hales
(17 September 1677–4 January 1761)

He was an English clergyman who made major contributions to a range of scientific fields including botany pneumatic chemistry and physiology. Stephen Hales made measurements of blood pressure in several animal species by inserting fine tubes into arteries and measuring the height to which the column of blood rose.

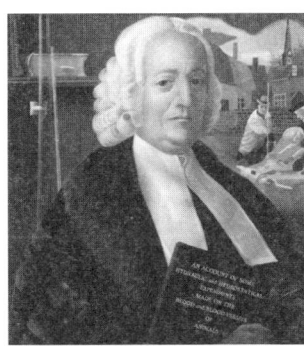

Stephen Hales

Scipione Riva Rocci
(7 August 1863 in Almese, Piedmont–
15 March 1937 in Rapallo)

He was an Italian internist and pediatrician who was a native of Almese. He earned his medical degree in 1888 from the University of Turin, and from 1900 until 1928 was director of the hospital in Varese. He is credited with developing an easy to use version of the sphygmomanometer.

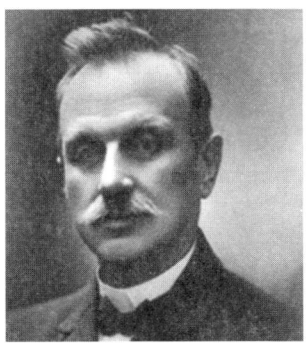

Scipione Riva Rocci

RECENT UPDATES

Digital Blood Pressure Monitor

The battery operated, palm top with LCD display screen digital blood pressure monitor is widely being used to monitor BP by patients or general public at home apart from it use by the practitioners. The cuff is wrapped around the upper arm. The pressure rises and then lowers and the arterial pressure and pulse reading appears on the screen. The pressure measuring ranges from 0 to 280 mmHg.

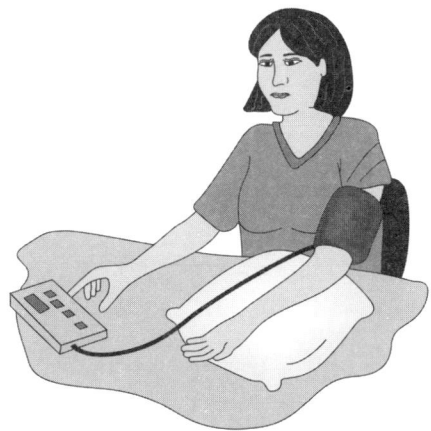

Exhibit 11.4 Digital blood pressure monitoring

How to Use a Home-based Blood Pressure Monitor?

Simple Steps to an Accurate Reading

There are a few simple steps that you can follow to be sure that you get an accurate reading of your blood pressure.

Before you take your blood pressure reading

1. Wear loose-fitting clothes like a short sleeved t-shirt so that you can push your sleeve up comfortably.
2. Before you take your readings, rest for 5 minutes. You should be sitting down in a quiet place, preferably at a desk or table, with your arm resting on a firm surface and your feet flat on the floor.
3. Make sure your arm is supported and that the cuff around your arm is at the same level as your heart. You may need to support your arm with a cushion to be sure it is at the correct height. Your arm should be relaxed, not tensed.
4. When you are taking your reading, keep still and silent. Moving and talking can affect your reading.
5. Take two or three readings, each about 2 minutes apart, and then work out the average. Some people find that their first reading is much higher than the next readings. If this is true for you, keep taking readings until they level out and stop falling, then use this as your reading.

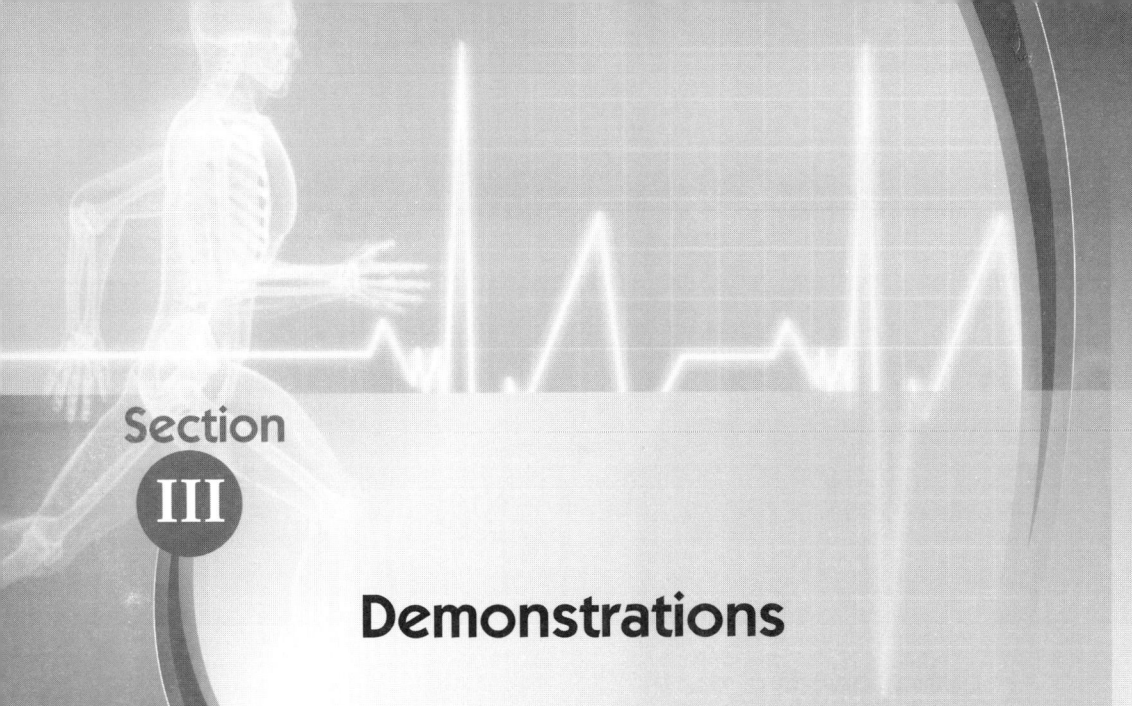

Section

III

Demonstrations

- ◆ Determination of erythrocyte sedimentation rate and packed cell volume
- ◆ Determination of specific gravity of blood
- ◆ Determination of osmotic fragility of red blood cells
- ◆ Determination of vital capacity and timed vital capacity
- ◆ Skeletal muscle experiments
- ◆ Electrocardiography: Demonstration of recording of normal electrocardiogram
- ◆ Clinical examination of respiratory system
- ◆ Clinical examination of cardiovascular system

12

Determination of Erythrocyte Sedimentation Rate and Packed Cell Volume

INTRODUCTION

Erythrocyte sedimentation rate is a simple nonspecific screening test that indirectly measures the presence of inflammation in the body. It measures the time taken for red blood cells to settle in a vertical tube. ESR exhibits the tendency of red blood cells to settle more rapidly in certain disease states, usually because of increases in plasma fibrinogen, immunoglobulins and other acute phase reaction proteins. The changes in red cell shape or numbers may also affect the ESR.

The hematocrit also known as PCV or erythrocyte volume fraction (EVF) is the volume percentage of red blood cells in blood. It is normally about 45% for men and 40% for women.

Aim: To determine the ESR of the given sample of blood.

THEORY

ESR is the rate at which RBCs settle down when blood to which an anticoagulant is added is allowed to stand in a specially designed narrow tube for 1 hour. The ESR is expressed in mm of clear plasma at the end of 1 hour.

The sedimentation occurs in three different stages:

Stage I : Rouleaux formation (piling of RBCs) and aggregation occurs in 10 minutes. Rouleaux formation is determined largely by increased levels of plasma fibrinogen and globulins.

Stage II : Sinking of the aggregates takes place at approximately 40 minutes.

Stage III: The aggregated cells pack at the bottom of the tube. This takes a period of 10 minutes

METHODS

ESR can be determined by Wintrobe's and Westergren's methods.

Wintrobe's Method

Materials and chemicals: Wintrobe's hematocrit tube with rack, anticoagulant mixture of potassium ammonium oxalate and Pasteur pipette, spirit, cotton and syringe with 22 gauze needle.

Wintrobe's hematocrit tube: It is a cylindrical tube approximately 11 cm in length with an internal bore of 2.5 mm. The tube is graduated in mm in both directions from 0 to 10 cm. The markings 0–10 from above downward are used for recording the ESR and markings 0–10 from below upward are used for recording hematocrit (PCV).

Procedures
1. Withdraw 5 mL of blood in penicillin bottle containing the anticoagulated powered mixture of double oxalate (6 mg of ammonium oxalate and 4 mg of potassium oxalate) and gently shake the bottle.
2. Draw the blood with the Pasteur pipette and introduce the tip of the pipette right down up to the bottom of the Wintrobe's tube.
3. Empty the blood slowly out of the pipette into hematocrit tube, taking care to avoid air bubbles.
4. The Wintrobe's tube is filled with blood up to the "0" mark and place the Wintrobe's tube vertically in its rack. At the end of 1 hour note the reading of clear plasma in the Wintrobe's tube.

Result

The ESR by the Wintrobe's method is _____ mm at the end of the first hour.

Normal values (Wintrobe's method): Males: 0–9 mm at the end of the first hour and females: 0–20 mm at the the end of the first hour.

Westergren's Method

Materials and chemicals: 3.8% sodium citrate solution as anticoagulant. Westergren's tube with rack, spirit, cotton and syringe with 22 gauze needle.

Descriptions: Westergren's tube is 300 mm in length, opened at both ends and has an internal diameter of 2.5 mm. It is graduated marking from 0 to 200 mm along the lower two-thirds of its length. The tube is held vertically in the Westergren's stand which is provided with rubber corks at the lower end and metal clips at the upper end so that tube is held vertically.

Procedures

1 Take 1 mL of 3.8% sodium citrate solution in penicillin bottle and add 4 mL of blood and then mix it gently.

2 Suck the citrated blood into the Westergren's tube up to the "0" mark and close the upper end with the finger immediately to prevent the blood from running out.

3 Press the lower end tightly on the rubber cork of the Westergren's stand and fix the tube vertically with the clip at the upper end.

4. Take the ESR reading at the end of 1 hour.

Result

The ESR by the Westergren's method is _____ mm at the end of 1 hour.

Normal values (Westergren's method): Males: 3–5 mm at the end of the first hour and females: 4–7 mm at the end of the first hour.

PACKED CELL VOLUME (Hematocrit)

Wintrobe's Method

1. Draw the venous blood and pour it in a penicillin bottle containing powder of double oxalate mixture. The Wintrobe's tube is filled with this anticoagulated blood up to 10 mark of the hematocrit readings.

2. Close the mouth of the tube with a cork and place the tube in the centrifuge machine.

3. Centrifuge the blood for 30 minutes at 3,000 revolution per minutes. Watch till cells settle down at bottom.

   Three layers are observed in the Wintrobe's tube.

   (a) Clear plasma above

   (b) Red layer below of the RBCs

   (c) Buffy layer in between of WBCs and platelets.

4. Remove the tube from centrifuge and not the reading of PCV (hematocrit) value from the tube. The height of column of RBCs is taken as PCV. Express the value as percentage of the blood.

Normal values (Wintrobes's method): Adult men: Average 45% (range 40–50%) and adult women: Average 42% (range 37–47%)

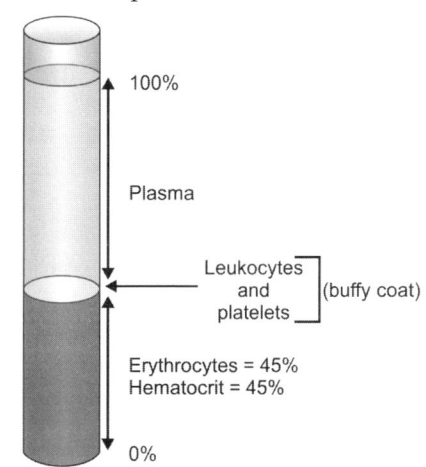

Fig. 12.1 Hematocrit, buffy coat and plasma

PRECAUTIONS

1. Take dry clean glass apparatus like tubes, pipette, dropper, etc for experiment.
2. The drawn venous blood should be immediately transferred into the penicillin bottle to prevent hemolysis.
3. Take note of the time of fixing the tube/pipette and of observed readings exactly after 1 hour.

DENTAL IMPLICATION

Raised ESR, C reactive protein (CRP) and plasma viscosity (PV) levels are all markers of inflammation. ESR, CRP and PV may increase in many inflammatory conditions in dental diseases causing periodontitis, gingivitis, dental cavities, dental abscess, pulpitis, impacted tooth, etc.

OBJECTIVE STRUCTURED PRACTICAL EXAMINATION (OSPE) QUESTIONS

1. **Enlist the causes of increase or decrease in ESR.**

Ans. The ESR is increased in anemia, acute or chronic infections, malignancies, nephrosis, etc. The ESR is decreased in polycythemia, leukemia, congestive heart failure, burns, dehydration, severe allergic reactions, etc.

2. **Enlist the conditions where PCV is increased and decreased.**

Ans. The causes of increased packed cell volume are polycythemia, congestive heart failure, burns and dehydration. Packed cell volume is decreased in anemia, bone marrow depression and severe leukopenia.

3. **Identify the instrument shown in the picture.**

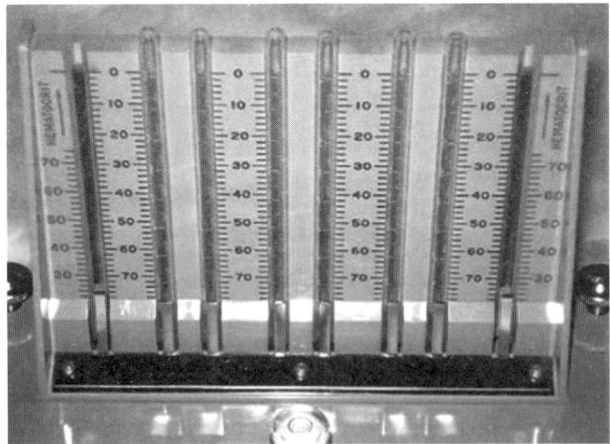

Fig. 12.2 Wintrobe's sedimentation rack

Ans. The instrument is Wintrobe's sedimentation rack.

4. **Read the results from the photo shown below.**

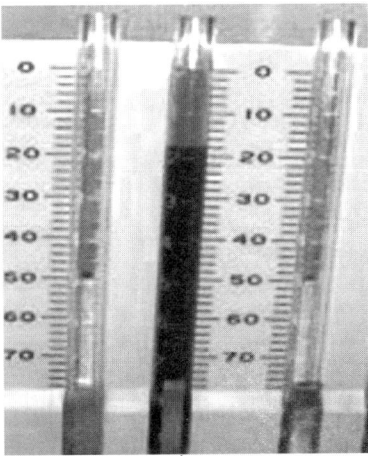

Fig. 12.3 ESR being measured by Wintrobe's tube

Ans. The photo shows ESR value of 18 mm at the end of 1 hour by Wintrobe's method.

VIVA QUESTIONS

1. **Define ESR. What are the factors which affect ESR?**

Ans. The rate at which the red blood cells settle down is known as erythrocyte sedimentation rate.

ESR depends on the shape, size and number of RBCs, temperature, tendency for rouleaux formation, plasma viscosity, length, diameter and position of ESR tubes and the anticoagulant used for the procedure.

2. **Name the two methods used to assess the ESR.**

Ans. Westergren's and Wintrobe's methods are used to assess the ESR

3. **What is the effect of temperature on ESR?**

Ans. The increase in temperature decreases the viscosity of blood and hence increases the ESR.

4. **Mention the clinical importance of performing the erythrocyte sedimentation rate.**

Ans. The high values of ESR indicate the presence of acute inflammatory reaction in the body and it also serves as a prognostic indicator for various diseases.

5. **Mention any two pathological causes for raised ESR.**

Ans. Hereditary spherocytosis and tuberculosis.

6. **Define hematocrit. Mention the different methods for measuring the hematocrit.**

Ans. Hematocrit or packed cell volume (PCV) is defined as the percentage of the volume (or parts) of blood occupied by the red cells.

The different methods for measuring PCV includes: (a) Macrohematocrit method, (b) microhematocrit method and (c) automated method

7. **What is the clinical significance of assessing the packed cell volume?**

Ans. The percentage of error associated with PCV method is less when compared to the hemoglobin estimation or red cell count. Hence, PCV is a more accurate test to determine the presence of anemia or polycythemia. It is also used in the calculation of various red cell indices.

8. **What are the advantages of microhematocrit method?**

Ans. The procedure is easy, cheap, less time consuming and requires very less quantity of blood when compared to the macrohematocrit method. The procedure is very useful in mass screening for anemia.

9. **How do you calculate the 'true' hematocrit or true cell volume?**

Ans. 'True' hematocrit or true cell volume is calculated by multiplying the hematocrit value obtained with 0.98.

10. **Why is the hematocrit of venous blood more than that of arterial blood?**

Ans. The red cells in venous blood contain higher concentration of chloride ions when compared to the red cells of arterial blood due to the mechanism of chloride shift. Since chloride ions are osmotically active particles, water enters into the red cells leading to increase in the size of these cells. Hence, the hematocrit of venous blood is more than that of the arterial blood.

MULTIPLE CHOICE QUESTIONS

1. **The following conditions are characterised by raised ESR, except**
   A. Pregnancy
   B. Leukemia
   C. Anemia
   D. Polycythemia

2. **Which among the following statements regarding ESR is correct?**
   A. ESR is done routinely to diagnose various pathological conditions
   B. ESR is high in polycythemia
   C. ESR does not depend on the nature of anticoagulant used
   D. ESR helps in assessing the prognosis of various diseases

3. **The following statements regarding Westergren's method are true, except**
   A. It is more sensitive than Wintrobe's method.
   B. Sodium citrate is the anticoagulant used in Westergren's method
   C. The Westergren's tube can also be used to measure packed cell volume
   D. Westergren's method is very useful in conditions characterised by high ESR values

4. **The following statements regarding Wintrobe's method are incorrect, except**
   A. It is more sensitive than Westergren's method
   B. Wintrobe's tube cannot be used to assess packed cell volume
   C. Sodium citrate is the preferred anticoagulant in Wintrobe's method
   D. Cannot be used in cases where ESR is grossly elevated

5. **Which among the following decreases the ESR?**
   A. Acute phase proteins
   B. Increase in temperature
   C. Anemia
   D. Afibrinogenemia

6. **The following conditions are characterised by increased PCV, except**
   A. Newborns
   B. Severe dehydration
   C. Pregnancy
   D. Polycythemia

7. **Which among the following is incorrect regarding PCV?**
   A. PCV of venous blood is lesser than the PCV of arterial blood
   B. PCV of females is lesser than the PCV of males
   C. The Wintrobe tube used for PCV determination can also be used to determine ESR
   D. PCV is more accurate than red cell count and hemoglobin estimation

8. **The following statements about Wintrobe's method of estimation of PCV are true, except**
   A. Hematocrit value is read from the scale marked from 0 to 10 from below upwards on the Wintrobe's tube
   B. Heparin is the preferred anticoagulant for Wintrobe's method of estimation of PCV.
   C. Prolonged centrifugation of the blood sample may result in mechanical damage to the red cell membrane leading to hemolysis
   D. PCV must be assessed within 6 hours of collection of the blood sample

Answers:

1 D	2 D	3 C	4 D	5 D	6 C	7 A	8 B

HISTORICAL ASPECT

Edmund Faustyn Biernacki (1866–1911)

Edmund Faustyn Biernacki (born on December 19, 1866 in Opoczno—died on December 29, 1911 in Lwów) was a Polish physician. He was the first one to note a relationship between the sedimentation rate of red blood cells in a human blood sample and the general condition of the organism. This method, known as the Biernacki reaction, is used worldwide to assess erythrocyte sedimentation rate (ESR).

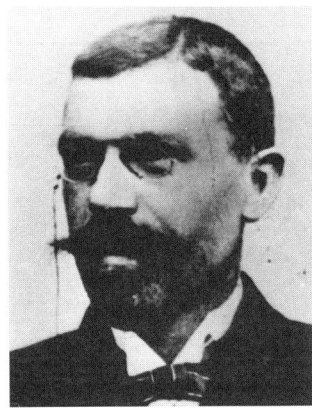

Edmund Faustyn Biernacki

RECENT UPDATES

1. Dengue fever is an acute viral illness and may affect children and adults. It can also progress to a severe form known as dengue hemorrhagic fever (DHF). Disease is transmitted through the bite of the infected mosquitoes of the genus *Aedes*. The high hematocrit value in dengue fever increases risk of dengue shock syndrome. The hematocrit levels are kept under observations for a minimum of 24 hours period. A hematocrit level elevated more than 20% of the normal range suggests hemoconcentration, especially after treatment with intravenous fluids and these finding precedes shock.

2. Professional athletes' hematocrit levels are measured as part of tests for erythropoietin (EPO) use or blood doping. The level of hematocrit is compared with the long-term level for that athlete taking into consideration individual variations in hematocrit level, and against an absolute permitted maximum.

3. Anabolic androgenic steroid (AAS) use can also increase the amount of RBCs and thus affects the hematocrit particularly in persons addicted to the compounds boldenone and oxymetholone.

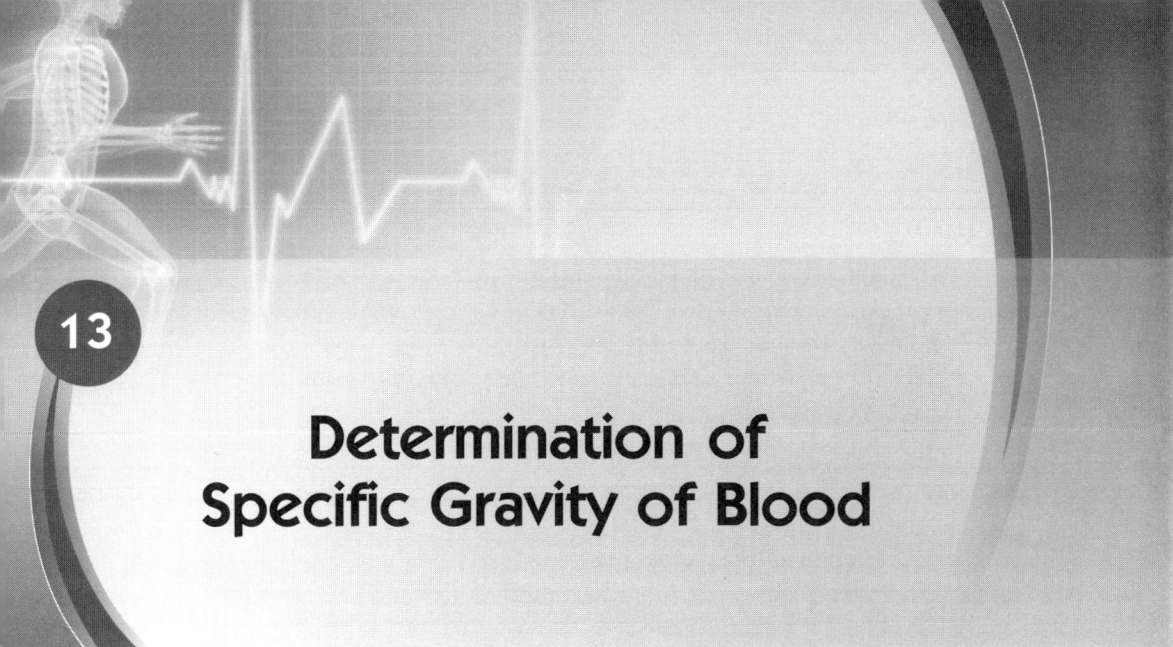

13

Determination of
Specific Gravity of Blood

Learning Objectives

The medical students should be able to:
1. Define the term specific gravity and tell the normal range of specific gravity of blood in humans.
2. Enlist physiological and pathological conditions which alter the specific gravity of blood.

INTRODUCTION

Specific gravity is defined as the mass of any volume of substance by mass of equal volume of water at 4°C (the density of water is the maximum at 4°C). The specific gravity is affected by alteration in red blood cell count; hemoglobin concentration; decreased plasma protein level, increase in water content, in pregnancy or in pathological conditions like vomiting and diarrhea.

The specific gravity (SG) of the provided blood sample is determined by the following methods:

I. **Direct method:** Take equal volume of blood and water in capillary tubes and weighed. The specific gravity of blood is determined as ratio of their weights.

II. **Indirect method:** Philips and Vanslykes $CuSO_4$ method.

Materials and chemicals: Distilled water, test tubes, dropper and stock solution of copper sulphate ($CuSO_4$) of specific gravity 1.100.

Principle: Specific gravity of blood is compared with solutions of $CuSO_4$ of known specific gravities. The specific gravity of the solution in which blood drop shall remain suspended for 15–20 seconds is the specific gravity of the blood.

Methods

1. Mix the distilled water with stock solution of $CuSO_4$ (10 mL of $CuSO_4$ solution is added proportionately to distilled water) so as to prepare $CuSO_4$ stock solution of specific gravity (SG) ranging from 1.050 to 1.066.

2. Add a drop of blood into each solution of the nine test tube serially from a height of about 1 cm with the help of a pipette.

3. Carefully observe the blood drop in the solution. If it is heavier than the solution, it will sink; and if it is lighter than the solution, it will float on the surface of the solution.

Table 13.1 Dilution principle for preparation of $CuSO_4$ solution of varying specific gravity (SG)

Test tube	1	2	3	4	5	6	7	8	9
$CuSO_4$ solution (mL)	4.9	5.1	5.3	5.5	5.7	5.9	6.1	6.3	6.5
Distilled water (mL)	5.1	4.9	4.7	4.5	4.3	4.1	3.9	3.7	3.5
SG of solution	1.050	1.052	1.054	1.056	1.058	1.060	1.062	1.064	1.066

Observe for the specific gravity of the solution in which blood drop remains suspended for 15–20 seconds. This will give the specific gravity of the blood sample. Due to covering of copper proteinate layer, blood drop remains suspended in the $CuSO_4$ solution as it is stable for about 15–20 seconds.

Normal values

- SG of blood: 1.048–1.066
- SG of RBCs: 1.092–1.095
- SG of plasma: 1.026–1.035

Hammer Schlag's Method

Note the equalizing density of two miscible liquids like chloroform (specific gravity 1.470) and benzene (specific gravity 0.88) to that of blood and this will be the specific gravity of the blood sample.

DENTAL IMPLICATION

Specific gravity measures the hemoglobin content and PCV. It is generally estimated as a parameter in research project and not done routinely. As specific gravity indicates blood proteins status and degree of dehydration; the measurement of specific gravity of blood will help to confirm physiological homeostasis state of patient prior to any dental surgery.

OBJECTIVE STRUCTURED PRACTICAL EXAMINATION (OSPE) QUESTIONS

1. **What is the normal range of specific gravity of blood? Compare the specific gravity of plasma with specific gravity of RBC.**

Ans. Specific gravity of plasma is 1.026–1.035. The specific gravity of RBC is 1.092–1.095.

2. **Enlist the conditions in which the specific gravity of blood is altered.**

Ans. Specific gravity of blood is low in anemia (decreased RBC count and hemoglobin concentration), hypoproteinemia (decreased plasma proteins), overhydration (after high water intake) and pregnancy.

    Specific gravity is high due to loss of fluid as in condition of vomiting and diarrhea.

Calculation

1. **Calculate the hemoglobin content and packed cell volume (PCV) of patient whose specific gravity of plasma is 1.030 and specific gravity of blood is 1.060.**

Ans. Hemoglobin content for 100 mL of blood

$$= \frac{33.9 \text{ (specific gravity of blood – specific gravity of plasma)}}{\text{(1.097– specific gravity of plasma)}}$$

$$= \frac{33.9 \ (1.060 - 1.030)}{(1.097 - 1.030)}$$

The hemoglobin concentration of patient is 14.6 gm%.

$$PCV = \frac{100 \text{ (specific gravity of blood – specific gravity of plasma)}}{(1.097 - \text{specific gravity of plasma})}$$

$$PCV = \frac{100 \ (1.060 - 1.030)}{(1.097 - 1.030)}$$

The PCV of patient is 45%.

VIVA QUESTIONS

1. **Define specific gravity.**

Ans. Specific gravity is the ratio of weight of a given volume of a fluid to the weight of the same volume of distilled water measured at $25°C$.

2. **Enlist the condition in which specific gravity increases.**

Ans. The specific gravity increases in the following conditions:

    a. Excessive fluid loss such as in vomiting, diarrhea and severe dehydration.

    b. Loss of plasma in burns leading to hemoconcentration.

    c. Polycythemia in residents of high altitude, patients of polycythemia vera, newborns, etc.

3. **Enlist the condition in which specific gravity decreases.**

Ans. The specific gravity decreases in the conditions such as anemia, pregnancy, renal diseases, starvation and malnutrition (decrease in plasma protein), in patients having intravenous fluid transfusions, etc.

4. **Name the common method employed for estimation of specific gravity of blood and plasma.**

Ans. The copper sulphate drop falling method is commonly used for the assessment of specific gravity of blood and plasma.

5. **Explain the correlation between the specific gravity of blood and hemoglobin levels.**

Ans. Specific gravity of blood is directly proportional to the amount of hemoglobin concentration. The blood sample with a hemoglobin level of 12.5 g/dL has a specific gravity of 1.053 g/mL.

MULTIPLE CHOICE QUESTIONS

1. **The average specific gravity of normal human erythrocytes is**
   A. 1.097   **B.** 1.030
   C. 1.050   **D.** 1.010

2. **The traditional method being used for donor screening at many blood centres**
   A. Copper sulphate specific gravity method
   B. Magnesium sulphate specific gravity method
   C. Potassium sulphate specific gravity method
   D. Sodium copper sulphate specific gravity method

Answers:

1 A	2 A

HISTORICAL ASPECT

Donald D. Van Slyke (1883–1971)

Donald D. Van Slyke received his BA and PhD degrees in chemistry at the University of Michigan. During World War II, a group of scientists at the Rockefeller Hospital led by Donald D. Van Slyke (1883–1971) devised a simple test for estimating blood volume by copper sulfate test in shock victims before and after a plasma infusion. The technique was tested clinically by a colleague stationed at the United States Typhus Commission Unit at the Cairo Fever Hospital in Egypt.

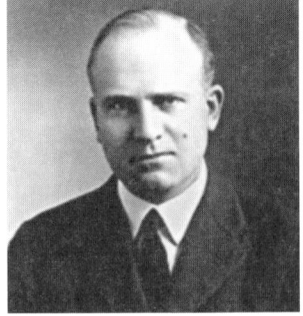

Donald D. Van Slyke

RECENT UPDATES

The blood fractionation is the process of separating it into its component parts. This is achieved by centrifuging the blood. An effective isolation of the cells affects immune monitoring and aids in better therapeutic care delivery.

The degree of separation of constituent cell layers in human blood by centrifugation can be enhanced by decreasing the natural water content of the red blood cells to increase the density or specific gravity of these red blood cells. Thereby red cell layer packs more tightly and also separates more completely from the next lighter cell layer of the granulocyte layer by use of potassium oxalate for selectively altering the specific gravity of the red blood cell constituent. The main reason for considering potassium oxalate for the above purpose is its dual use of its excellent ability to desirably alter the specific gravity of the red blood cell types and also its anticoagulant role.

Potassium oxalate is used in concentration of about 200 mg/dL of solution merely for its anticoagulant function while its concentration in the range of about 400 mg/dL to about 600 mg/dL solution provides the required degree of cell separation.

14

Determination of Osmotic Fragility of Red Blood Cells

INTRODUCTION

The ease with which the RBCs are hemolyzed in hypotonic solution is called osmotic fragility of RBCs. It is expressed in terms of concentration of hypotonic solution in which the cells are getting hemolyzed.

PRINCIPLE

1. The RBCs when get placed in isotonic solution, i.e. solution with same tonicity as that of plasma (e.g. 0.9% sodium chloride; 5% glucose; 10% mannitol and 20% urea solution), they remain suspended in it. They neither swell nor shrink because the osmotic pressure of the isotonic solution is equal to the osmotic pressure within the RBCs.
2. However, RBCs when placed in hypotonic solution (e.g. <0.9% sodium chloride), they absorb water from outside and get swelled and finally burst.
3. When RBCs placed in hypertonic solution (e.g. >0.9% sodium chloride), the fluid within the RBC goes out of cells and they shrink.

Aim: To study the osmotic fragility of RBCs.

Matarials and chemicals: Lancet, cotton, spirit, a set of clean test tubes, test tube rack, distilled water, freshly prepared 1% nail solution, pipette (2 mL) and dropper.

Procedures

1. Place the test tubes in the rack and number them serially from 1 to 12.
2. Prepare hypotonic solutions of various strengths by mixing the required number of drops of 1% sodium chloride solution and distilled water in the test tubes 1–12, as given in Table 14.1.

Table 14.1 Procedure for preparation of increasing hypotonicity of sodium chloride solution

Test tube Nos.	1	2	3	4	5	6	7	8	9	10	11	12
No. of drops of distilled water added	3	9	10	11	12	13	14	15	16	17	18	25
No. of drops of 1% NaCl added	22	16	15	14	13	12	11	10	9	8	7	0
Percentage of saline solution	0.88	0.64	0.60	0.56	0.52	0.48	0.44	0.40	0.36	0.32	0.28	0

> **Note** that the first tube contains nearly isotonic saline and that the last tube contains distilled water (tonicity-nil).

3. The tubes are to be shaken well and then add a drop of blood in each tube.
4. Mix the blood with saline by inverting each tube gently.
5. After 1 hour, observe the tubes against a white background.
6. Take care not to shake the tubes.
7. Note the percentage of sodium chloride in the tube which shows the beginning of hemolysis and the percentage of sodium chloride in the first tube that shows complete hemolysis.
8. The clear, straw-colored, supernatant fluid indicates absence of hemolysis with unhemolyzed RBCs settled at the bottom.
9. A tube with partial hemolysis will show a pink colored upper supernatant fluid proportionate to the extent of hemolysis and a layer of unhemolyzed RBCs at the bottom of the tube.
10. Complete hemolysis is confirmed by a uniformly pink colored solution with no RBCs at the bottom.

Results: Record your observations and results as given below.

1. Beginning of hemolysis occurs in _____ % saline.
2. Complete hemolysis of cells is seen in _____ % saline.
3. The osmotic fragility of RBCs ranges from _____ % to _____ % saline.
4. Compare your results with the fragility range for normal RBCs and interpret.

PRECAUTIONS

1. Prepare hypotonic solutions of various strengths by mixing the required number of drops of 1% sodium chloride solution and distilled water carefully.
2. After adding blood, test tube should not be shaken vigorously for mixing purpose, otherwise mechanical hemolysis may occur.
3. Wait for 1 hour to observe complete hemolysis.

SIGNIFICANCE

1. In normal healthy individuals, osmotic fragility of RBC begins in 0.48% sodium chloride and ends in 0.34% sodium chloride solution.
2. RBCs osmotic fragility increases when they become spherical, e.g. in spherocytosis (independent of the cause). It begins in 0.7% sodium chloride and ends in 0.45% sodium chloride solution.
3. RBC's osmotic fragility is decreased when they become slender, e.g. in iron deficiency anemia and thalassemia. It begins in 0.36% sodium chloride and ends in 0.24% sodium chloride solution.

DENTAL IMPLICATION

• Research studies with determination of osmotic fragility of RBC can be carried out in dental patients having thalassemia, sickle-cell anemia or iron deficiency anemia.

It should also be remembered that hemolyzed RBCs cause increased release of hemoglobin which gets metabolized to bilirubin producing hemolytic jaundice, if urine is acidic and GFR is slow, the hemoglobin which passes through glomeruli is precipitated in the tubules as acid hematin. This obstructs the lumen of tubules producing renal tubular damage. Later, anuria sets in resulting in renal failure.

OBJECTIVE STRUCTURED PRACTICAL EXAMINATION (OSPE) QUESTIONS

Non-skilled Questions

1. **What does osmotic fragility test signify?**

Ans. The osmotic fragility test is a measure of the resistance of erythrocytes to hemolysis by osmotic stress. The test consists of exposing red cells to varying strengths of hypotonic saline solutions and measuring the degree of hemolysis by colorimeter at room temperature.

2. **State the principle of osmotic fragility test.**

Ans. The principle of the test is that the normal RBC is able to resist the influx of water to a limited extent. When the cells are placed in a hypotonic solution, the RBC absorbs water due to osmotic pressure and leads to swelling of RBC. In hypertonic solution the RBC shrinks.

OSPE for Practice

1. Perform the osmotic fragility test and record your observations.

2. Add a drop of the given sample of blood to the test tube containing urea solution and record your observation.

3. Add a drop of the given sample of blood to the test tube containing 10% sucrose solution and record your observation.

4. Add a drop of the given sample of blood to the test tube containing 5% dextrose solution and record your observation.

VIVA QUESTIONS

1. What is the normal range of osmotic fragility of red cells?

Ans. Hemolysis begins at 0.45 to 0.50% saline and completes at about 0.30–0.33% saline.

2. What would you observe if the red cells are suspended in a solution containing 10% glucose?

Ans. Since 10% glucose is a hypertonic solution, water moves out from the red cells into the surrounding medium resulting in shrinkage of the red cells.

3. List a few conditions characterised by increased red cell fragility.

Ans. Conditions such as hereditary spherocytosis, congenital/autoimmune hemolytic anemia and G6PD deficiency are characterised by increased red cell fragility.

4. List a few conditions characterised by decreased red cell fragility.

Ans. Conditions such as iron deficiency anemia, thalassemia, sickle cell anemia and acholuric jaundice are characterised by decreased red cell fragility.

5. Mention the clinical significance of osmotic fragility test.

Ans. Osmotic fragility test is used as a screening tool for hereditary spherocytosis.

6. List the factors which affect the osmotic fragility of red cells.

Ans. Permeability of red cell membrane and red cell surface to volume ratio are the factors which affect the osmotic fragility of red blood cells.

MULTIPLE CHOICE QUESTIONS

1. Which of the following is true regarding osmotic fragility of red cells?

    A. Osmotic fragility begins at 0.60 to 0.56 and completes at 0.48 to 0.44% saline

    B. Osmotic fragility begins at 0.64 to 0.60 and completes at 0.48 to 0.44% saline

    C. Osmotic fragility begins at 0.45 to 0.50 and completes at 0.30 to 0.33% saline

    D. Osmotic fragility begins at 0.56 to 0.52 and completes at 0.30 to 0.33% saline

2. The following conditions are characterised by decreased osmotic fragility, except
   A. Iron deficiency anemia
   B. Sickle cell anemia
   C. Thalassemia
   D. Hereditary spherocytosis

3. Red blood cells when suspended in hypertonic solution will undergo
   A. Cell swelling
   B. Cell shrinkage
   C. No change in size
   D. None of the above

4. Suspension of red cells in the following solutions can result in hemolysis, except
   A. 5% Dextrose
   B. Urea solution
   C. Hypotonic saline
   D. None of the above

5. Increased red cell fragility is seen in
   A. Obstructive jaundice
   B. Iron deficiency anemia
   C. Hereditary spherocytosis
   D. Thalassemia

Answers:

1 C	2 D	3 B	4 A	5 C

RECENT UPDATES

The microfluidic chip-based system for measuring the osmotic fragility of RBCs is made from a Y-shaped polydimethylsiloxane (PDMS) micro channel sealed to a glass cover plate. The different degrees of hemolysis (no hemolysis, partial hemolysis, and complete hemolysis) are estimated with this platform. This device provides a definitive screening platform for diseases marked by RBC abnormalities; and also aids differential diagnosis with great simplicity, high speed and minimal requirement of blood samples.

15

Determination of Vital Capacity and Timed Vital Capacity

Learning Objectives

After learning the practicals, the students should be able to:

1. Understand the procedure of spirometry for recording of vital capacity and timed vital capacity.
2. Explain the indication and significance for carrying spirometry.
3. Evaluate the type of respiratory disorder (obstructive or restrictive) from the findings.

INTRODUCTION

Spirometer is used to evaluate lung volume and capacity which stands immensely helpful in diagnosis of respiratory disorders. Spirometry is indicated for diagnosis and management of asthma, detection of respiratory disease in patients presenting with symptoms of breathlessness, measuring bronchial responsiveness in patients suspected of having asthma, diagnosis and differentiation between obstructive lung disease and restrictive lung disease, assessment of impairment from occupational asthma and conducting preoperative risk assessment before anesthesia or cardiothoracic surgery.

Though the prime aim of teaching this practical is to determine vital capacity and timed vital capacity, the normal lung volumes are also discussed for better understanding of the applied respiratory physiology.

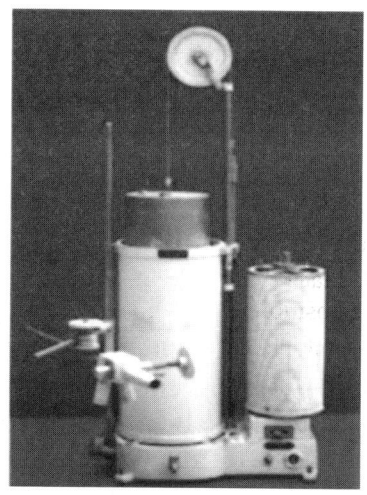

Fig. 15.1 Spirometer and vitalograph

127

Aim: Determination of vital capacity and timed vital capacity.

Instruments: Benedict-Roth's spirometer and vitalograph.

METHODS

Recording of lung volumes and capacities: The subject is asked to sit comfortably.

1. After familiarizing the subject with the mouthpiece; close the nostril of the subject with nose clip.
2. Ask the subject to breathe from the atmosphere for 1–2 minutes.
3. Turn the three way connectors so that the subject can breathe the air under the spirometer bell.
4. Adjust the spirometer speed at 2 mm/second.
5. Record the normal breathing for a minute to calculate the tidal volume, the respiratory rate and the resting pulmonary ventilation.
6. The subject should be asked to take a maximal inspiration after a normal expiration and the tracing for the same is recorded. Calculate the inspiratory capacity and the inspiratory reserve volume from the graph.
7. Ask the subject to make maximal expiration following normal inspiration. Use this to compute the expiratory reserve volume.
8. Ask the subject to make a maximal expiration after a maximal inspiration. This gives the vital capacity.
9. The graphical record which is obtained is the spirogram.
10. The speed of the spirometer is set at the rate of 20 mm per second.
11. Ask the subject to take a maximal inspiration and then to make a maximal expiration quickly. Record this to compute the timed vital capacity [forced expiratory volume (FEV)].
12. Calculate the volume of air expired in 1st, 2nd and 3rd seconds. This will give the FEV1, FEV2 and FEV3. Express these volumes as a percentage of the vital capacity.

Recording of Vital Capacity using the Vitalometer

The vitalometer has a structure similar to the basic structure of the Benedict-Roth's spirometer. The vital capacity values can be read off directly from its graduated pulley (dial).

1. Place the spirometer vertical and adjust the spirometer bell and set it at its lowest position. Now set the pointer on the dial to the zero mark.
2. Ask the subject to sit comfortably on the examination stool.
3. Ask the subject to take a maximal inspiration from the atmosphere.
4. Apply the noseclip and asked the subject to breathe out maximally into the spirometer through the mouthpiece.
5. Note the reading on the dial. Repeat the procedure three times at intervals of 2 minutes. Report the maximum value as the vital capacity.

Results

Tidal volume _____ mL.

Vital capacity _____ mL.

FEV1 _____ mL (_____%).

OBJECTIVE STRUCTURED PRACTICAL EXAMINATION (OSPE) QUESTIONS

1. **Study the graph and define the various lung volumes and capacity as shown in Fig. 15.2.**

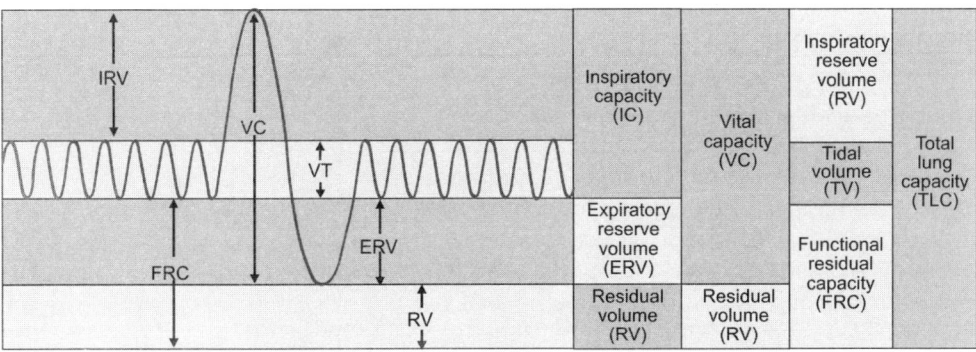

Fig. 15.2 Graph showing lung volume and capacity

Ans. The various lung volumes as shown in the graph are:

- Tidal volume (TV): It is the amount of air inspired during normal, relaxed breathing. It is about 500 mL.
- Inspiratory reserve volume (IRV): It is the maximum amount of air which can be inhaled after the inspiration of a normal TV. It is about 1,100 mL.
- Expiratory reserve volume (ERV): It is the maximum amount of air which can be exhaled after the expiration of a normal TV. It is about 1,200 mL.
- Residual volume (RV): It is the volume of air still remaining in the lungs after the expiratory reserve volume is exhaled. It is about 1,200 mL.

Summing specific lung volumes produces the following lung capacities:

- Total lung capacity (TLC) is the maximum volume of air present in the lungs (TLC = TV + IRV + ERV + RV). It is about 6,000 mL.
- The vital capacity (VC) about 4,800 mL is the total amount of air that can be expired after fully inhaling (VC = TV + IRV + ERV = approximately 80% TLC). The value varies according to age and body size.

- Inspiratory capacity (IC): It is the maximum amount of air that can be inspired (IC = TV + IRV). It is about 3,600 mL.
- The functional residual capacity (FRC): It is the amount of air remaining in the lungs after a normal expiration (FRC = RV + ERV). It is about 2,400 mL.

2. **Describe the indicators of timed vital capacity.**

Ans. The important indicators of timed vital capacity are FVC, FEV1 and FEV1%.

Forced Vital Capacity

Forced vital capacity (FVC) is the volume of air that can forcibly be blown out after full inspiration. It is measured in liters.

Forced Expiratory Volume in 1 Second

Forced expiratory volume in 1 second (FEV1) is the volume of air that can forcibly be blown out in 1 second after full inspiration.

FEV1/FVC RATIO (FEV1%)

FEV1/FVC (FEV1%) is the ratio of FEV1 to FVC. In healthy adults, it is approximately 75–80%. FEV1 is diminished because of increased airway resistance to expiratory flow in obstructive diseases (asthma, COPD, chronic bronchitis and emphysema). In restrictive diseases (pulmonary fibrosis), the FEV1 and FVC are reduced proportionally and the value may be normal or even increased as a result of decreased lung compliance.

A derived value of FEV1% is FEV1% predicted which is defined as FEV1% of the patient divided by the average FEV1% in the population for any person of similar age, sex and body composition.

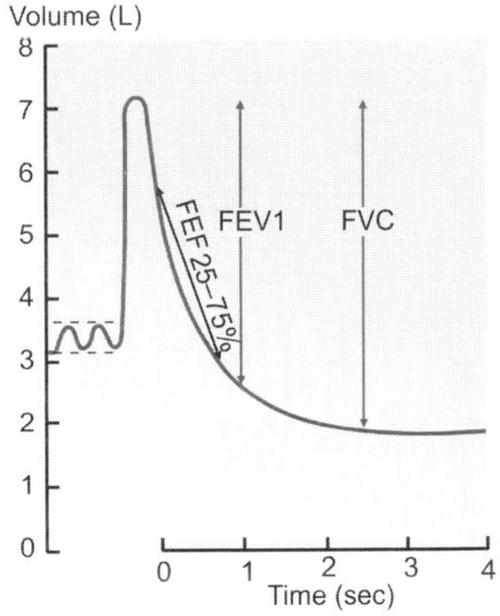

The FEF 25–75% is also known as MMEF (maximum mid-expiratory flow) is the average expiratory flow over the middle half of forced vital capacity (FVC). Reduced MMEF indicates small airway disease.

Fig. 15.3 FEV 1% recording

OBJECTIVE STRUCTURED PRACTICAL EXAMINATION (OSPE) QUESTIONS

1. **Record your forced volume vital capacity (FVC).**

Ans.
- Asked the subject for examination to take deep breath, and then exhale into the sensor as hard as possible. (Yes/No)
- The soft nose clips is used to pinch the noise to prevent air escaping through the nose. (Yes/No)
- Observing manoeuvre of patient ensuring that it is performed for at least 6 seconds. (Yes/No)
- Noting the reading of the spirometer. (Yes/No)

2. **Measure vital capacity by collecting the air in spirometer.**

Ans. • Bring the bell to its lowest position by gently pushing it down;   (Yes/No)
adjusts pointer needle at zero.

• After breathing normally for a minute, inspires deeply and   (Yes/No)
fully and after closing the nostrils with thumb and finger and
mouthpiece held firmly between the lips exhales the air with
maximum effort forcefully.

• Note the reading.

VIVA QUESTIONS

1. **Define vital capacity.**

Ans. Vital capacity is the maximum amount of air a person can expel from the lungs
after a maximum inhalation. It is equal to the sum of inspiratory reserve volume,
tidal volume, and expiratory reserve volume.

2. **What is the range for normal adult vital capacity?**

Ans. A normal adult has a vital capacity between 3 and 5 litres.

3. **Which device is used for measuring lung volume and capacity?**

Ans. The lung volume and capacity can be measured using a device known as a
spirometer.

4. **Define functional residual capacity (FRC).**

Ans. Functional residual capacity (FRC) is the volume of air that remains in the lungs
during quite breathing. FRC = ERV + RV.

5. **Which are the conditions in which restrictive lung disease occur?**

Ans. The conditions in which restrictive lung disease occur are fibrosing alveolitis,
severe scoliosis, ankylosing spondylitis, and even in weakness of the respiratory
muscles (e.g. myasthenia gravis, Guillain Barre syndrome and phrenic nerve
palsy).

MULTIPLE CHOICE QUESTIONS

1. **The tidal volume (TV) is about**
   A. 500 mL   B. 300 mL
   C. 400 mL   D. 700 mL

2. **The inspiratory reserve volume (IRV) is about**
   A. 3100 mL   B. 3900 mL
   C. 4000 mL   D. 5700 mL

3. **The expiratory reserve volume (ERV) is about**
   A. 1,200 mL
   B. 300 mL
   C. 400 mL
   D. 700 mL

4. **Residual volume (RV) is about**
   A. 500 mL
   B. 1200 mL
   C. 400 mL
   D. 700 mL

5. **The total lung capacity (TLC) is about**
   A. 6000 mL
   B. 3000 mL
   C. 2000 mL
   D. 1000 mL

Answers:

| 1 A | 2 A | 3 A | 4 B | 5 A |

HISTORICAL ASPECT

John Hutchinson (1811–1861 AD)

John Hutchinson, a surgeon, had begun his work with spirometers. He invented the spirometer to measure vital capacity and he believed it to be a powerful indicator of longevity. His spirometer consisted of a calibrated bell inverted in water which captured exhaled air from the lungs. Hutchinson recorded the vital capacities of over 4,000 persons with his spirometer. Hutchinson's water spirometer is still used today with a few alterations which include the reduction of the mass of the bell and the addition of graphic and timing devices.

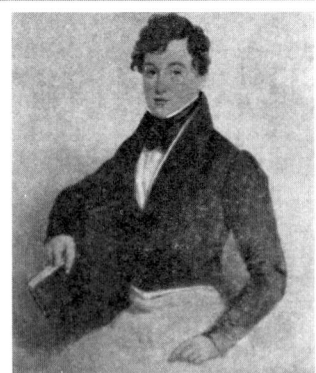

John Hutchinson

RECENT UPDATES

The spirometry test is performed using a computerized device called a computerized spirometer.

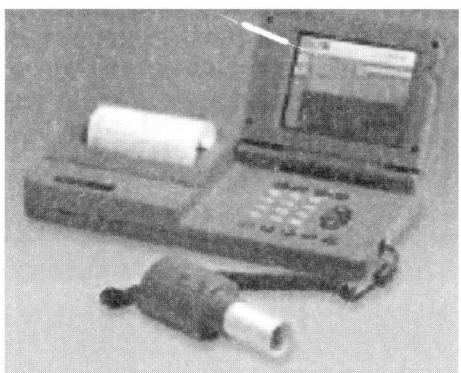

Exhibit 15.1 Computerised spirometer

PROCEDURES

The patient is asked to take the deepest breath they can, and then exhale into the sensor completely and forcefully for. During the test, soft nose clips may be used to prevent air escaping through the nose. Sterilized filter mouthpieces must be used to prevent the spread of any infection. The computerized readings are obtained for lung capacity.

LIMITATIONS OF TEST

The maneuver is dependent on patient cooperation and effort and is normally repeated at least three times to ensure reproducibility. As results are dependent on patient cooperation, FVC can only be underestimated, never overestimated.

Skeletal Muscle Experiments

EXPERIMENT 1: AN INTRODUCTION TO THE AMPHIBIAN EXPERIMENTS

Introduction

The main aim of the amphibian experiments is to study the response of a living tissue to an external stimulus. The prerequisite to conduct this experiment includes living tissue preparation, a stimulating device and a recording device. Frogs are used to demonstrate the physiological aspect of the nerve muscle physiology. The nerve muscle preparation obtained from frog is adequate for survival under average experimental conditions hence being used in physiological studies.

Stimulating device: The types of stimuli which can be used for experimentation are mechanical, chemical, electrical, thermal, etc.

But the electrical stimulus as being least injurious to tissue and as its intensity frequency, duration and timing being easily controlled is preferable mode for stimuli response.

Recording device: The response is recorded using a writing lever (provided with a capillary pen ink writer at its tip) which inscribes on the surface of a moving drum mounted on a kymograph.

Kymograph (power supply): It has an electric motor which works on power supply of 220 volt AC, and it rotates a vertical shaft. A speed selector is set at desired speed of rotation as required. The kymograph can be driven at speed between 0.12 mm/sec and 640 mm/sec. Select the neutral position denoted by "N", to rotate the vertical shaft manually. The rotation can be abruptly started or stopped by a clutch. The cylindrical drum pasted with recording paper is fixed to the vertical shaft. Two projecting contact arms are present at the base of the shaft. As these arms make contact with the contact block the electrical circuit is completed and the electrical stimulus passes to the tissue.

Du Bois Raymond induction coil converts the available low voltage, high ampere, direct (continuous current) into induced current of short duration. It is made up of primary and the secondary coils having insulated

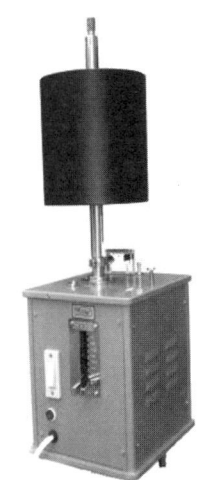

Fig. 16.1 Kymograph

copper wire wound round a soft iron core. The primary coil has 3,000 turns and the secondary coil has 5,000 turns. The primary coil terminals are connected to the DC source and the secondary coil terminals are connected to the electrodes. Nearer the secondary coil is to the primary; stronger is the current induced in the secondary.

When the two coils are parallel the induced current is strongest, weaker when they are at an angle.

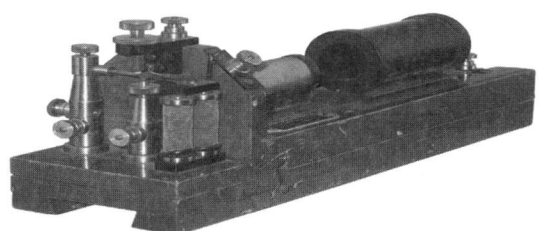

Fig. 16.2 Du Bois Raymond induction coil

Simply key or primary key is used for opening or closing the primary circuit. The short-circuiting key or secondary key is connected in parallel in the secondary circuit and is kept closed for preventing accidental passage of the induced current flowing to the tissue. **Tap key** is used to make or break the circuit by pressing the key gently and releasing it suddenly. It is connected in series with the low voltage mains in the primary circuit.

Neef's hammer is built-in automatic interrupter connected in series with the primary coil of the induction coil. It interrupts the primary circuit about 40 times.

Vibrating variable interrupter enables more accurate interruption of the primary circuit at a much lower frequency (up to 25/sec) than the Neef's hammer.

Electronic stimulator: The electrical stimulus is provided using the electronic student stimulator. It works on 220 V AC power supply. The stimulator carries a mode switch which can be set in either of the three positions, namely EXT, SINGLE and REPEAT.

In the EXT position, the stimulus is delivered to the tissue particularly as the contact arms on the vertical shaft make contact with the contact knob of the kymograph.

In the SINGLE position, a single stimulus can be delivered to the tissue, particularly by pressing and releasing the SINGLE button.

In the REPEAT position, multiple stimuli can be delivered to the tissue at the desired frequency which is to be set by adjusting the frequency knob.

The stimulus duration as required can be set at 0.5 ms or 1.5 ms by adjusting a toggle switch provided. A glowing bulb indicates that the electrical stimulus is available. The stimulus is transmitted to the tissue by connecting the OUT terminals of the stimulator to the stimulating electrodes.

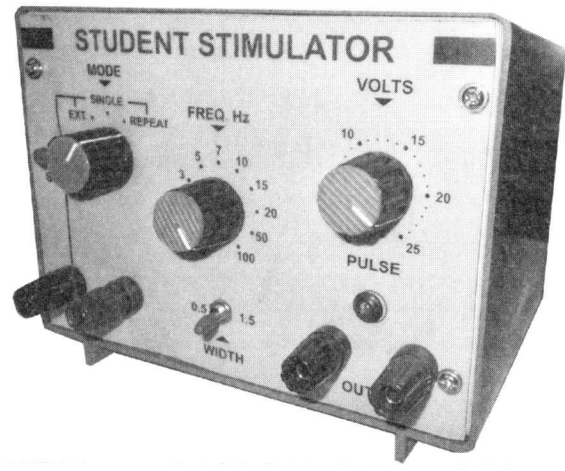

Fig. 16.3 Student stimulator

Stimulating electrode: It consists of two metallic hooks, each of which has a ball and socket arrangement. A perspex block holds the two metallic hooks. This is generally used in skeletal muscle experiments.

Muscle trough: It is made of perspex or plastic. The trough holds the isolated nerve muscle preparation as it is kept immersed in a nutritive solution. It carries the stimulating electrode on one side and a writing lever on the other side. The floor of the trough has a cork to which the nerve muscle preparation can be fixed. A drainage tube is attached to the floor of the muscle trough.

Myograph stand: It is made of a heavy base to which a vertical rod is attached. The rod rotates on its vertical axis smoothly. The muscle trough is fixed to the vertical rod of the myograph stand.

Writing lever: It consists of a narrow metallic plate to which a long thin metal wire carrying a writing pen is attached. The narrow plate is attached to a metallic fulcrum rod and this carries a hook. As screw can prevent the downward movement of the hook, it is called the after loading screw. The writing lever mounts on one side of the muscle trough. A small weight (10 g) is suspended from the writing lever and is 2 cm from the fulcrum.

Tuning fork (100 Hz): The tuning fork with a frequency of 100 vibrations per second is used for the nerve muscle experiments.

Stimulus marker (signal marker): It consists of an electromagnet and a writing lever. Whenever the stimulus is applied to the tissue, the electromagnet gets magnetized and pulls the writing lever down. Thus, the time of the application of the stimulus is marked.

EXPERIMENT 2: NERVE MUSCLE PREPARATION

Aim: Dissecting a gastrocnemius muscle sciatic nerve preparation in the frog.

Instruments and chemicals: Stunning rod, pithing needle, scissors, forceps, glass rod and amphibian Ringer's solution.

Animal species: Frog

Procedures
1. Give a firm blow on the head of the frog with the stunning rod.
2. Insert the pithing needle inside the vertebral canal and skull so as to destroy the spinal cord and the brain. This procedure is called pithing.
3. Place the frog on its back on a dissection board.
4. Take a scissor and cut the skin of the frog around its middle; and remove the skin off the lower limbs using toothed forcep.
5. Lift the urostyle with blunt end forceps and cut the pelvic girdle on either side, taking precaution that the underlying sciatic nerves are not damaged. Identify the insertion roots of the sciatic nerves.
6. Incise the vertebral column above and below the roots of the sciatic nerves. Cautiously separate the isolated segment of the vertebral column into two by cutting it in-between.
7. The sciatic nerve is to be isolated and exposed with a blunt glass rod.
8. Trace the sciatic nerve from the thigh muscles up to knee joint and remove all adhesions.
9. Identify the gastrocnemius muscle and free the muscle from the tibia. Separate its tendon from the ankle joint and tie a piece of thread to the tendon.
10. Cut the tibia below the knee joint and the femur above the knee joint taking care not to cut the sciatic nerve.
11. Isolate the nerve muscle preparation. Keep the nerve muscle preparation immersed in the amphibian Ringer's solution till it is needed for the experiment.

Composition of Amphibian Ringer's Solution

Sodium chloride: 0.6%

Potassium chloride: 0.014%

Calcium chloride: 0.012%

Sodium bicarbonate: 0.02%

Sodium biophosphate: 0.001%

EXPERIMENT 3: SIMPLE MUSCLE CURVE

Aim: To record the simple muscle curve in an isolated skeletal muscle by giving a single electrical stimulus to the nerve supplying the muscle.

Instruments and chemicals: Stunning rod, pithing needle, scissors, forceps, student stimulator, muscle trough, writing lever, stimulating electrode, kymograph, recording drum, tuning fork (100 Hz) and amphibian Ringer's solution.

Procedures

1. Isolate and make a gastrocnemius muscle nerve preparation ready.
2. Placed it in the muscle trough. Pour the amphibian Ringer's solution into the muscle trough.
3. Fix the knee joint with a pin to the cork base of the muscle trough.
4. Pull and attach the thread from the tendon to the hook of the writing lever.
5. Check whether the after loading screw touches the hook. Ideally, a 10 g weight can be suspended from the hole of the writing lever around 2 cm from the fulcrum.
6. Hold the vertebral piece with forcep and place the nerve on the stimulating electrode.
7. The EXT position on the student stimulator is to be selected for operation. The EXT terminals are connected to the terminals of the contact knob of the kymograph.
8. Connect the OUT terminals of the stimulator with the stimulating electrode.
9. Switch on the stimulator. Rotate the vertical rod of the myograph stand ensuring that the writing lever does not touch the drum.
10. Switch on the kymograph and allow it to rotate at the fastest speed (640 mm/sec) by turning the clutch to the vertical position. Increase the voltage gradually from the stimulator till a muscle twitch of 3–4 cm height is observed. Stop the kymograph by turning the clutch to horizontal position.
11. Rotate the vertical rod of the myograph stand and make the writing lever now touch the drum.
12. Rotate the drum manually and make the contact arms touch the contact knob of the contact block. At this position, mark a vertical line on drum in order to indicate the point of stimulation.
13. Start the kymograph and record a simple muscle curve.

14. Label the point of stimulus (PS), the latent period (LP), contraction period (CP) and relaxation period (RP) on the simple muscle curve.

15. Allow the kymograph to rotate at the same speed (640 mm/sec). Using a tuning fork of 100 Hz, take a time tracing below the simple muscle curve.

16. Calculate the duration of the latent period, the contraction period and the relaxation period from the simple muscle curve.

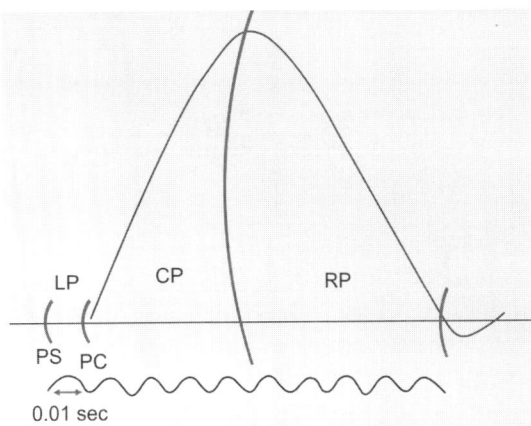

Fig. 16.4 Simple muscle twitch exhibiting latent period (LP), contraction period (CP) and relaxation period (RP)

Simple Muscle Twitch

Simple muscle twitch is the contraction and relaxation of muscle following a single stimulus. The different phases of the simple muscle curve as shown in Fig. 16.4 are:

- **Latent period (LP):** It represents the period from the point of stimulus to the onset of contraction. The normal duration of latent period is 0.01–0.012 second. The latent period is due to the time taken for the transmission of impulse along the nerve fiber to the muscle, neuromuscular delay, time taken for excitation contraction coupling and also due to inertia of lever.

- **Contraction period (CP):** It is the period between the point of contraction and the point of maximum contraction. The normal duration of contraction period is 0.04 second.

- **Relaxation period (RP):** It is the period between the point of maximum contraction and the point of relaxation of muscle. The normal duration of RP is 0.05–0.06 second.

EXPERIMENT 4: EFFECTS OF TWO SUCCESSIVE STIMULI ON SKELETAL MUSCLE CONTRACTION

Aim: To demonstrate the effects of two successive stimuli on skeletal muscle contraction.

Materials and instruments: Same as for recording simple muscle curve.

Method:

1. Arrange nerve muscle preparation and record the simple muscle twitch as explained in earlier practical of record of simple muscle curve.

2. The projecting strikers are separated slightly so that they strike the contact button in close succession. The distance between the strikers is so adjusted that a second stimulus should fall in the first half of the latent period of the simple muscle twitch of the first stimulus. The contraction is to be recorded using the same stimulus strength. The points of stimulation are to be marked.

3. The same procedure is repeated after progressively widening the distance between the strikers so as the second stimulus falls: In the second half of the latent period, in the contraction period, in the relaxation period and lastly immediately after the relaxation period.

Take the time tracing in the usual manner as explained in experiment of recording of simple muscle curve.

Inference

When two successive stimuli of maximal strength are induced to a skeletal muscle, the response to the second stimulus depends upon time when the second stimulus is given after the first stimulus.

1. If the second stimulus falls during the latent period of the muscle, the muscle is said to be completely refractory as there is no additional response. Refractory period is the period when second stimulus of adequate strength fails to produce a response. The refractory period in skeletal muscle is less than 0.005 second and it has two phases:

    (a) *Absolute refractory period:* It is the period during which a second stimulus does not produce a response irrespective of the intensity of the stimulus.

    (b) *Relative refractory period:* It is the period during which if a second stimulus of stronger intensity is provided; it produces a response.

2. If time of application of second stimulus falls during contraction or relaxation phase; second muscular response is there. When the second stimulus fall during contraction phase, the graph obtained shows increase in force of contraction, also called summation of contraction. When the second stimulus is applied during relaxation phase, the relaxation is arrested and another contraction results. This phenomenon is due to the beneficial effect because the second stimulus gets benefited by the changes produced in the muscle due to the first stimulus. The beneficial effect is due to release of more Ca^{2+} from sarcoplasmic reticulum, increase in the temperature of the muscle, decrease in internal viscosity and resistance of the muscle and decrease in the inertia of the recording system.

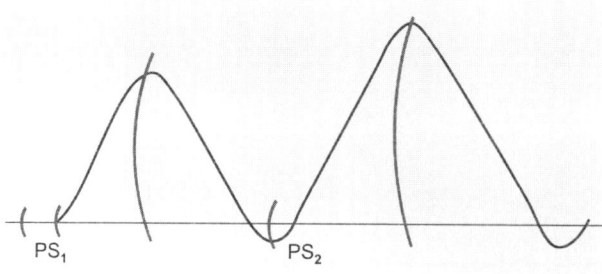

Fig. 16.5 Effect of second stimulus when induced after relaxation phase

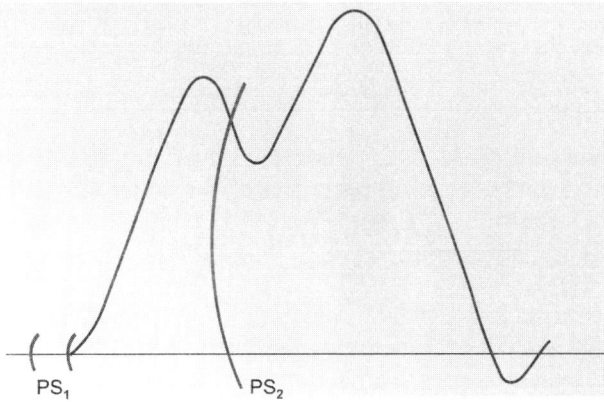

Fig. 16.6 Effect of second stimulus when induced during relaxation phase

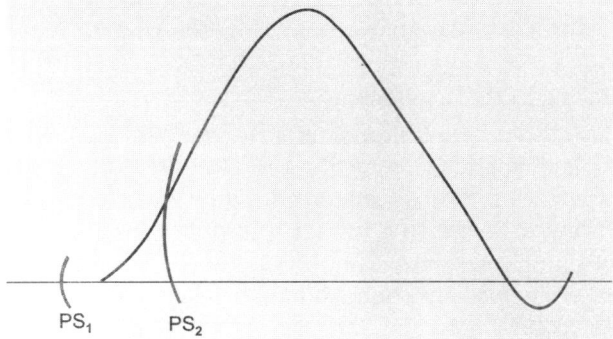

Fig. 16.7 Effect of second stimulus when induced during contraction phase

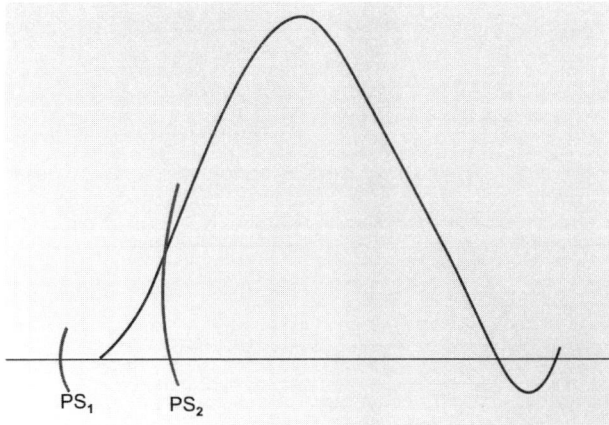

Fig. 16.8 Effect of second stimulus when induced during refractory period

EXPERIMENT 5: EFFECT OF TEMPERATURE ON SIMPLE MUSCLE TWITCH

Aim: To study the effect of temperature on simple muscle twitch.

Materials and instruments: Same as for recording simple muscle curve except that Lucas chamber is used in place of myograph board, thermometer and cold and warm amphibian Ringer's solution.

Method:
1. Arrange nerve muscle preparation; remember Lucas chamber is used in place of myograph board. Fill the chamber with amphibian Ringer's solution and record the simple muscle twitch using maximal stimulus as explained in earlier practical of simple muscle curve. Note the temperature of the Ringer solution.
2. Drain off the Ringer's solution and replace it with fresh hot Ringer's solution having temperature of about 40°C. Now without changing the strength of stimulus and using the same baseline and point of stimulus, record another simple muscle twitch.
3. Repeat the whole procedure using cold Ringer's solution having temperature of about 10°.
4. Take the time tracing in the usual manner.

The effect of warm Ringer's solution on muscle contractile response is exhibited as decrease duration of latent period, contraction period and relaxation period and increase in amplitude of contraction. Warm Ringer's solution raises the temperature of the muscle, hence reducing its inertia and the synaptic delays are minimized.

The effect of cold Ringer's solution on muscle contractile response is exhibited as increase latent period, increase in contraction and relaxation period and decrease in amplitude of muscle contraction.

This is due to decrease in enzymatic and metabolic processes, increase in viscosity of muscle protein and decrease in velocity of nerve conduction and transmission.

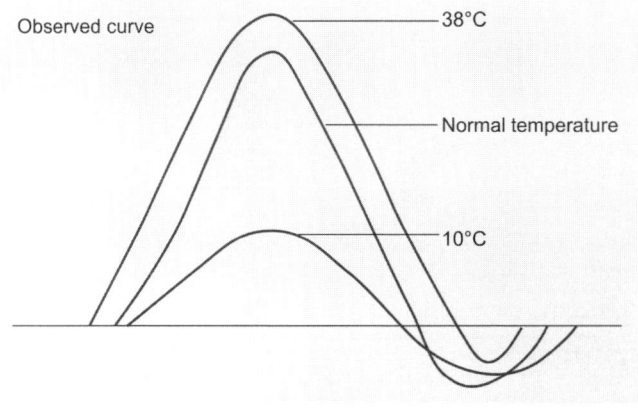

Fig. 16.9 Effect of temperature on simple muscle twitch

EXPERIMENT 6: GENESIS OF FATIGUE IN THE ISOLATED NERVE MUSCLE PREPARATION

Aim: Demonstration of genesis of fatigue in the frog's nerve muscle preparation.

Material and instrument: Same as for recording simple muscle curve.

Method:

1. Arrange nerve muscle preparation and record the simple muscle twitch as explained in earlier practical of record of simple muscle curve.
2. Record the first three simple muscle curves; stop the kymograph and label the three curves.
3. Remove the writing lever from the drum and allow the kymograph to rotate and the muscle to contract.
4. Apply the wirting lever to the drum and then record every 10th contraction till the muscle contractions cannot be recorded.
5. Take the time tracing below the simple muscle curves, close to the baseline.

Inference

Fatigue is defined as the inability of muscle to respond to a stimulus, any further even after repeated stimulation. When a muscle is repeatedly stimulated initially in the first few contractions, there is increase in amplitude due to beneficial effect; but when further stimulated, amplitude decreases and there is incomplete relaxation and finally the muscle does not respond to any further stimulation. The causes of fatigue are depletion of acetylcholine, accumulation of metabolic waste products like lactic acid and decrease store of glycogen and creatine phosphate. The synapse is the site of fatigue in an intact animal. Neuromuscular junction is the site of fatigue in an isolated preparation. The fatigue is quickened on by increased frequency of stimulation, increase in temperature or lack of O_2.

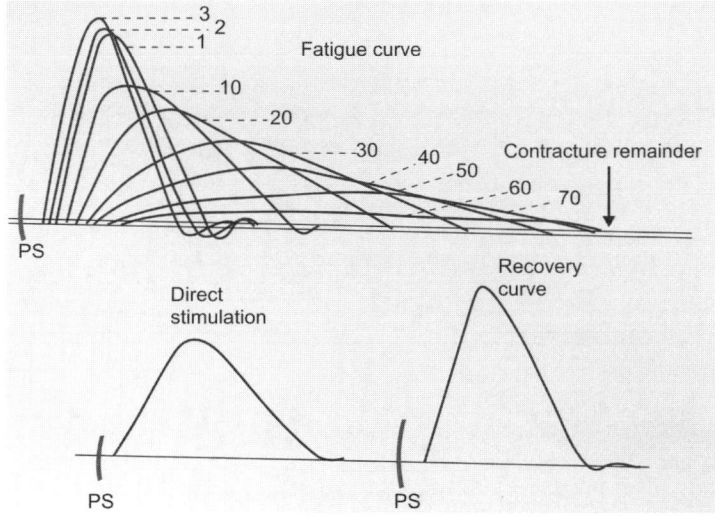

Fig. 16.10 Phenomenon of fatigue

EXPERIMENT 7: EFFECT OF INCREASING STRENGTH OF STIMULUS ON SKELETAL MUSCLE CONTRACTION

Aim: To study the effect of increasing strength of stimuli on skeletal muscle contraction.

Instruments and chemicals: Same as for simple muscle twitch recording.

Method:

1. Arrange the nerve muscle preparation as for recording a SMT except that the drum is not included and in its place an electromagnetic signal marker is included into the primary circuit in series.
2. The drum is placed in neutral gear and put in stationary position. The signal marker pointer is brought in conduct with the drum.
3. The primary key is kept closed and short circuiting key is opened. Move the secondary coil farthest away from the primary coil. Press tap-key briefly and then release it. The signal marker moves and marks the point of stimulus on the drum.

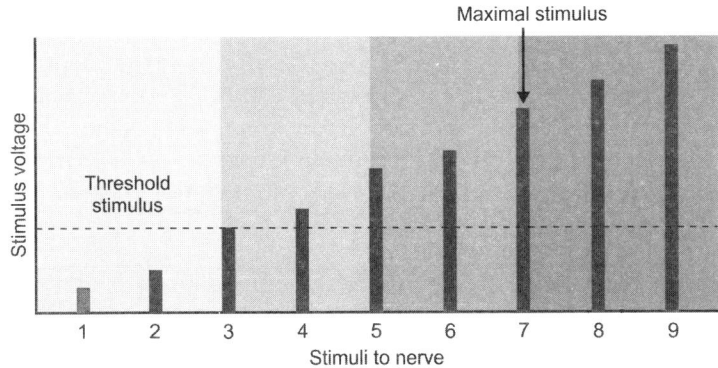

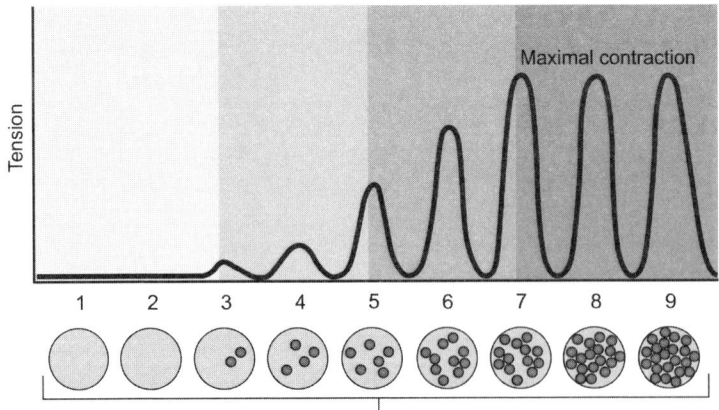

Fig. 16.11 Effect of increasing strength of stimulus on muscle contraction

4. Rotate the drum manually so that the pointer moves about 1 cm on the drum. Then move the secondary coil near the primary coil by 1 cm at a time and press the tap-key and release it. At every point, test the response of the muscle to make and break shock separately.

   (At least 15 sec. must elapse between make and break shocks to avoid beneficial effect. The distance is inversely related to the strength of the stimulus.)

5. Continue the experiment till further increase in the intensity of stimulus is without effect on the height of the contraction.

Inference

On giving a stimuli of subminimal strength, then there is no response. When the strength of stimulus increased, a response is produced and is the maximum at the maximal stimulus. The threshold of excitation of different motor neurons supplying a single skeletal muscle differs, therefore, with the increase in strength of stimulus, more and more motor units get recruited and thereby the height of contraction increases.

Hereafter even if supra-maximal stimulus is applied, there will be no increase in the response because by then all the motor-units have been activated. Gradation of muscle response depends on the optimal length of the muscle (the length at which they develop maximum active tension), number of motor units activated at a time and frequency of discharge in individual nerve fiber.

EXPERIMENT 8: GENESIS OF TETANUS

Aim: Effect of increasing frequency of stimuli on skeletal muscle contraction.

Instruments and chemicals: Same as for recording a simple muscle twitch, electromagnetic signal marker and variable interrupter.

Method:

1. The nerve muscle preparation is arranged similar to that for recording a simple muscle twitch. Exclude the drum from the circuit. Connect an electromagnetic single marker and a variable interrupter into the primary circuit in series.

2. Adjust the induction coil so that it delivers a maximal stimulus.

3. Set the variable interrupter into operation adjusting the vibrating rod to provide five stimuli per sec and start the drum at slow speed (12.5 mm/sec), open the short circuiting key to stimulate the muscle and after recording 5–6 contractions on the drum close it.

4. Increase the frequency of stimuli progressively to 10, 15, 20, 25, 30, 35 and 40 per sec and take a record of muscle response.

   (Neef's hammer may be included in the primary circuit in series as it enables the delivery of higher frequency of stimuli till the muscle tetanizes)

Inference

1. **Incomplete tetanus:** There is incomplete tetanus where subsequent stimuli fall during relaxation period of the previous one. So, the curves obtained will have a wavy appearance.

2. **Treppe or clonus:** This occurs at a frequency of 20 vibration/sec. There is partial fusion of individual contractions due to incomplete relaxation and as a result curves do not touch baseline. This is called clonus.

3. **Tetanus:** There is a smooth sustained contraction due to mechanical fusion of curves. Here subsequent stimuli fall during contraction period of previous one, but electrical properties are separated.

The minimum frequency at which tetanus occurs is called *critical fusion frequency.* In frog, it is 25 vibration/sec. The critical fusion frequency usually depends on duration of contraction period and it is inversely proportional to the contraction period. The conditions which increase the contraction period such as cold or fatigue will decrease the critical fusion frequency. At a frequency of 30 vibration/sec complete fusion of contractions take place, thereby producing a smooth sustained contraction called tetanus.

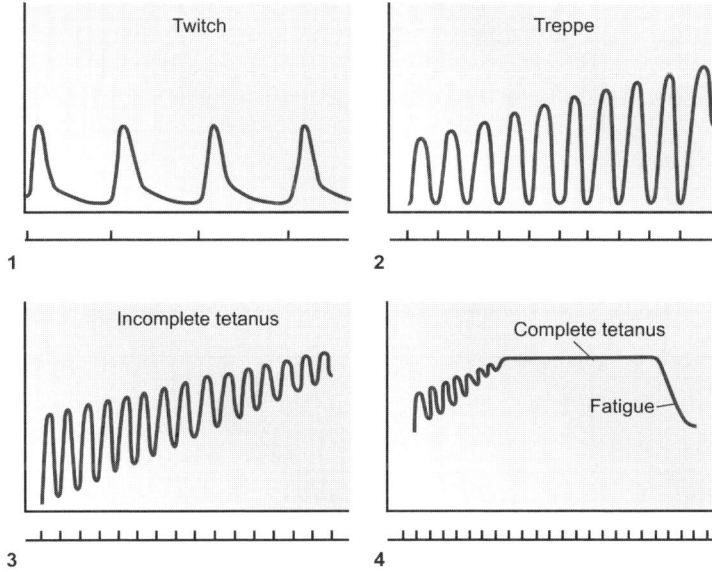

Fig. 16.12 Genesis of tetanus

EXPERIMENT 9: EFFECT OF AFTERLOAD AND FREELOAD ON MUSCLE CONTRACTION, CALCULATION OF WORK DONE

Aim: To demonstrate the effects of two successive stimuli on skeletal muscle contraction.

Materials and instruments: Same as for recording simple muscle curve and weight of 10 gm, 20 gm, 30 gm, 40 gm, 50 gm, 60 gm.

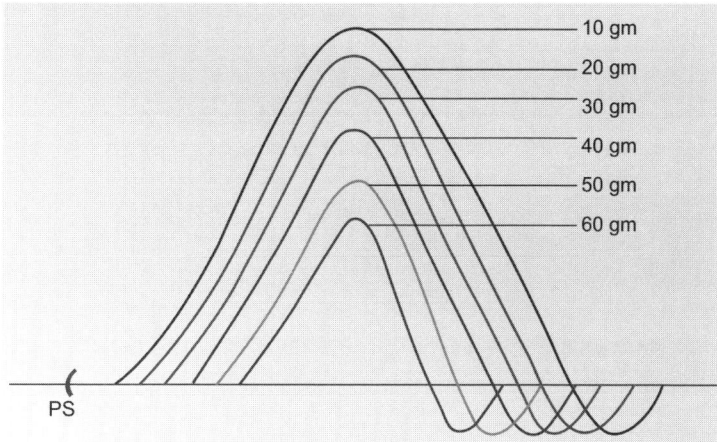

10 gm
20 gm
30 gm
40 gm
50 gm
60 gm

PS

Fig. 16.13 Effect of freeload and after load on muscle contraction

Method

1. Arrange nerve muscle preparation: Exclude the drum from the circuit. Record the simple muscle twitch as explained in the practical of effect of increasing strength of stimuli on skeletal muscle contraction.

2. Record in free loaded condition: Adjust the screw of fulcrum so that it does not touch the vertical arm of the writing lever and hang weight of 10 gm and record simple muscle twitch gradually increasing the weight up to 60 gm.

   Record in afterloaded condition: Adjust the screw of fulcrum so that it touches the vertical arm of the writing lever and hang weight of 10 gm and record simple muscle twitch gradually increasing the weight from 10 gm to 60 gm.

Theory

Afterload: The load acting on the muscle after it starts contracting is the afterload.

Freeload: The load acting on the muscle before it starts contracting is the freeload. The muscle fibers are stretched before it contracts.

Inference

As the load increases, the amplitude of contraction decreases. The contraction obtained for a given weight in preloaded or freeloaded condition is of higher amplitude than that obtained for the same weight in afterload because in freeload condition the initial length of the muscle is increased so there is increase in force of contraction. The Starling's law is applicable in this condition.

Calculation of Work Done

The force applied to move an object through a given distance is the work done by the muscle.

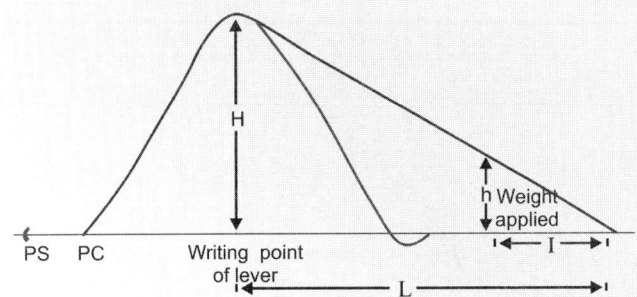

Fig. 16.14 Calculation of work done by studying the graph

$W = F \times h$

$$h = \frac{H \times I}{L}$$

Note:

W = Work done

F = Force applied

H = Apparent height of contraction for each weight applied

h = Actual height to which weight is lifted

I = Distance between fulcrum of lever and weight applied

L = Distance from the fulcrum to the writing lever

OBJECTIVE STRUCTURED PRACTICAL EXAMINATION (OSPE) QUESTIONS

Non-skilled OSPE Questions

1. **Identify the graph and interpret.**

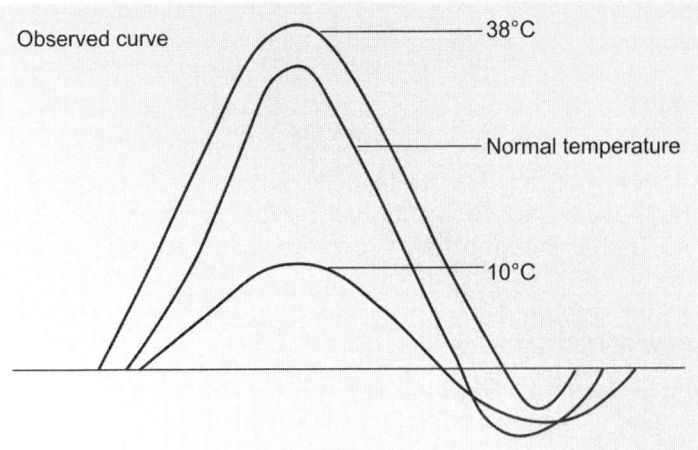

Ans. **Effect of temperature on simple muscle twitch**

The effect of warm Ringer solution on muscle contractile response is decreased in duration of latent period, contraction period and relaxation period and increased in amplitude of contraction as warm solution reduces its inertia and the synaptic delays are minimized. The effect of cold Ringer solution on muscle contractile response is exhibited as increase latent contraction and relaxation period and decrease in amplitude of muscle contraction attribute to decrease rate of enzymatic and metabolic processes, increase viscosity of muscle protein and decrease in velocity of nerve conduction.

2. **Define fatigue. What are its causes and enumerate the site of fatigue?**

Ans. Fatigue is defined as the inability of muscle to respond to a stimulus any further even after repeated stimulation. When a muscle is repeatedly stimulated, initially there is increase in amplitude in the first few contractions due to beneficial effect; but when further stimulated, amplitude decreases and there is incomplete relaxation. The causes of fatigue are depletion of acetylcholine, accumulation of metabolic waste products like lactic acid and decrease store of glycogen and creatine phosphate. The synapse is the site of fatigue in an intact animal. Neuromuscular junction is the site of fatigue in an isolated preparation.

VIVA QUESTIONS

1. **Describe the various types of muscles.**

Ans. The three types of muscles are:

A. *Skeletal muscle* is striated, the cells are unbranched and have multinucleate syncytia. These muscles are capable of voluntary and forceful contractions.

B. *Cardiac muscle* is striated, cells may be branched and have either mono- or binucleate cells. They are connected with one and other by *intercalated discs*. Cardiac muscle is capable of involuntary, strong and rhythmic contractions.

C. *Smooth muscle* is non-striated and found in the walls of the visceral organs having mononucleate cells. The smooth muscle cells synthesize collagen, elastin, and proteoglycans (like fibroblasts). These muscle cells are capable of relatively slow contractions.

2. **Enlist the basic units of muscle cell organization.**

Ans. The basic units of muscle cell organization are sarcolemma (plasmalemma of muscle cells), sarcoplasm (cytoplasm of muscle cells excluding the myofibrils), fascicle, perimysium, endomysium and epimysium.

3. **Describe the types of fatigue in human muscle.**

Ans. Muscle fatigue may be peripheral or central. The peripheral fatigue occurs due to exhaustion of energy reserves and accumulation of metabolic products in the active muscle while central fatigue which is subjective to central nervous system motivation mechanism and characterized by work-related pain in the involved muscles and joints that prevents the continuation of physical exercise or may decrease the persons motivation to continue the exercise.

4. What is the triad of skeletal muscle?

Ans. The T-tubule along with terminal cisternae on either side forms the triad in skeletal muscle.

MULTIPLE CHOICE QUESTIONS

1. Sarcomere is

 A. The portion of myofibril in between two Z lines.

 B. The portion of myofibril in between two I bands

 C. Contractile protein connected with Z disc and actin

 D. Contractile protein connected with M disc and myosin

2. Myosin I is present in

 A. Sperms   **B.** Serum

 C. Urine   **D.** Sweat

Answers:

 1 A 2 A

HISTORICAL ASPECT

Animal Experimentation

Francois Magendie (1783–1855)

Galen, the most noted physician of the Roman Empire, developed vivisection as a tool for methodical physiological investigation. He demonstrated the power of surgical interventions to produce a deeper understanding of bodily functions.

 Andreas Vesalius (1514–1564) revised the long-accepted anatomical system of Galen (as derived entirely from animal dissections) and encouraged experimental re-evaluation of Galenic theories of physiology as well. The most significant correction of Galen's physiology was accomplished by William Harvey (1578–1657), whose demonstration of the

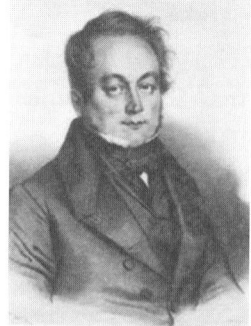

Francois Magendie

circulatory movement of the blood through the body was on observations of the contractions of the heart, ligation of the aorta and vena cava, and other vivisection procedures performed on about eighty species. Harvey's De Motu Cordis (1628) confirmed importance of animal experimentation as an invaluable technique for physiological discovery. Later even in early 1800, experimentation were approached to elucidate the physiological processes. Francois Magendie (1783–1855) during the period 1805 through the 1820s used animal experimentation to investigate and infer regarding such questions as the mode of action of strychnine, the mechanism of emesis, and the functioning of the nervous system.

Magendie insisted on analyzing function without being prejudiced by anatomical structure, and confirmed irrevocably the superiority of the experimental method for physiological in Francois Magendie (1783–1855).

RECENT UPDATES

Parvalbumin is a protein occuring in the cytosol of fast-twitch muscle fibers (type F). It accelerates muscle relaxation after brief contractions by binding cytosolic calcium in exchange for magnesium. Parvalbumins binding affinity for calcium is higher than that of troponin but lower than that of sarcoplasmic reticulum calcium ATPase. Therefore, it functions as a "slow" Ca^{2+} buffer.

The Di-Hydro Pyridine Receptor (DHPR) are arranged in rows and directly opposite to the rows of Ca^{2+} channels called ryanodine receptors (RYR1 in skeletal muscle) in the adjacent membrane of the SR. The RYR1 is associated with a DHPR and RYR1 open when they directly sense by mechanical means—a conformational change in the DHPR due to action potential. DHPR stimulation at a single site in skeletal muscle is enough to trigger the coordinated opening of an entire group of RYR1, thereby generating impulse transmission.

17

Electrocardiography: Demonstration of Recording of Normal Electrocardiogram

Learning Objectives

After completing the practicals, the students should be able to:

1. Understand electrophysiology of heart as it relates to electrocardiogram (ECG).
2. Understand the unipolar and bipolar methods of recording the ECG.
3. Identify the various waves of the ECG and student should be able to explain the causes for the waves, calculate heart rate, duration of each wave and RR and QT intervals.

INTRODUCTION

An ECG is the graphical record produced by an electrocardiograph (machine that records the electrical activity of the heart over time). ECG picks up electrical impulses generated by the polarizarion and depolarization of cardiac tissue and translates into a waveform. The waveform is then used to measure the rate and regularity of heartbeats, evaluate size and position of the chambers, identify underlying pathological cause of the heart and review the effects of drugs or devices used to regulate the heart such as a pacemaker.

Aim: Demonstrating the normal procedure of recording an ECG and training the student to acquire clinical skills to interpret a normal ECG.

PRINCIPLES

The electrical potentials which are generated by the heart are transmitted through the body. These potentials can be recorded from the body surface by placing electrodes at different positions over the body. Electrocardiograph picks up, amplify and record the potentials of the heart from the body surface. The graphic record of the electrical potentials of the heart is known as the "ECG".

ELECTROCARDIOGRAPH

A single channel electrocardiograph is used for recording an ECG. The instrument amplifies the electrical potentials as they are picked up by the electrodes placed over the body surface. These amplified potentials move a heated stylus which records the ECG on a wax coated heat sensitive paper. The speed of the moving paper can be either 25 or 50 mm/sec. The height of the vertical deflection of the stylus represents the voltage. The sensitivity may be adjusted to 1, 2 or 0.5 cm for 1 mV.

ECG Paper

ECG machines run at a standard rate (25 mm per second) and use paper with standard-sized squares. Each small square (1 mm) represents 40 ms (0.04 seconds), and each large square (5 mm) represents 200 ms (0.2 seconds). On the y-axis, each small square represents 0.1 mV.

ECG Leads

There are 12 leads in the standard surface ECG, three bipolar and nine unipolar. There are six unipolar leads placed on the chest and are called the chest leads, the three bipolar and three unipolar leads which are placed on the limbs are known as limb leads.

Chest Leads

Chest leads or precordial leads are unipolar leads that record the potential difference between an exploring electrode and a neutral electrode. The six precordial leads V_1–V_6 are positive electrodes placed at six different positions as follows:

V_1 : Fourth intercostal space on the right side of the sternum,

V_2 : Fourth intercostal space on the left of the sternum,

V_3 : Midway between V_2 and V_4,

V_4 : Fifth intercostal space in the mid-clavicular line,

V_5 : Fifth intercostal space in the anterior axillary line,

V_6 : Fifth intercostal space in the midaxillary line.

Limb Leads

The limb leads view the heart in a vertical plane called the frontal plane. Each lead has its own specific view of the heart at different angle.

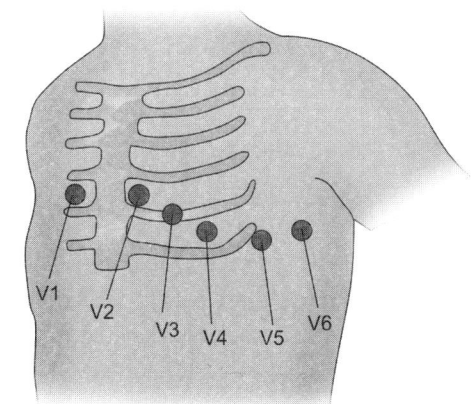

Fig. 17.1 Precordial leads

Bipolar Limb Leads

1. Lead I: Records the difference in potential between right arm (RA) and left arm (LA).

2. Lead II: Records the difference in potential between right arm (RA) and left leg (LL).
3. Lead III: Records the difference in potential between left arm (LA) and left leg (LL).

Unipolar Limb Leads

aVR—active (exploring) electrode on the right arm.

aVL—active (exploring) electrode on the left arm.

aVF—active (exploring) electrode on the left leg.

Leads aVR, aVL and aVF are augmented limb leads (named after their inventor Dr Emanuel Goldberger and are collectively known as the Goldberger's leads). Unipolar limb leads record the potential difference between one limb and a neutral electrode. The recording obtained from unipolar limb leads are small. Therefore, the augmented limb leads are generally used. These leads record electrical activity between the one lead and the other two limbs. The size of the potential is increased by 50% without changing the configuration of the record.

PROCEDURE FOR RECORDING AN ECG

1. Ask the subject to lie supine on the hospital bed or examination couch.
2. Clean the skin and apply ECG jelly for better contact.
3. Place electrodes on the flexor aspect of the left and right wrists and the left and right legs above the ankle.
4. Fasten the electrodes firmly to the skin by straps. The leads then must be placed correctly.
   The ECG leads should be placed as follows:
   a. LL: Left leg distally
   b. RL: Right leg distally
   c. LA: Left arm distally
   d. RA: Right arm distally
   e. V1: Fourth intercostal space to the right of the sternum
   f. V2: Fourth intercostal space to the left of the sternum
   g. V3: Midway between V2 and V4
   h. V4: Fifth left intercostal space along midclavicular line
   i. V5: At the horizontal level of V4 along anterior axillary line
   j. V6: At the horizontal level of V5 along midaxillary line.
5. The electrode on the right leg acts as the ground electrode.
6. Adjust the paper speed rate at 25 mm/sec. Center the writing pen.
7. Calibrate the voltage sensitivity such that 1 mV = 1 cm.
8. Connect the wires from the electrodes to the input socket of the ECG machine.
9. Record the ECG in each of the 12 leads as mentioned above using the lead selector.

Indications for performing an ECG include:
1. Irregular heart rate or palpitations
2. Chest pain
3. Increased heart rates (>100 bpm)
4. Decreased heart rates (<50 bpm)
5. Collapse or syncope (collapse with spontaneous return of consciousness)
6. Chest trauma where cardiac injury is suspected, for example, blunt trauma to the chest (as might occur when a pedestrian is struck by car)
7. Preoperative assessment of at-risk patients (for example, the elderly, patients of hypertension, diabetes mellitus, renal diseases, metabolic disorders, etc)

Results

Note the observation in the format given below.

Name of the voltage component (mV)	*Duration (sec)*
P wave	
QRS complex	
T wave	
PR segment	
ST segment	
PR interval	
QT interval	
Heart rate/minute	

Calculation of heart rate from RR interval of the ECG

At a paper speed of 25 mm/sec.

$$\text{Heart rate} = \frac{60 \text{ sec} \times 25 \text{ mm}}{\text{RR interval (mm)}} = \frac{1,500 \text{ (mm)}}{\text{RR interval (mm)}}$$

DENTAL IMPLICATION

As a dental surgeon one has to manage patients of oral diseases having preexisting systemic diseases. Hence before conducting any dental procedure or dental surgery, it is advisable to have an ECG recorded and physician consultation for planning treatment protocol. The clinical condition in which ECG is indicated to include myocardial infarction, pulmonary embolism, cardiac murmurs, syncope or collapse, seizures and cardiac dysrhythmias. Moreover, the dental surgeons while treating patients with systemic disease or while operating should monitor ECG during anesthesia and surgery. If any characteristic changes are seen on electrocardiography like pathological Q waves or sudden development of ST elevation or depression while in dental clinic or indoor, immediate assistance should be addressed to a general physician for management of myocardial infarction.

OBJECTIVE STRUCTURED CLINICAL EXAMINATION (OSCE) QUESTIONS

Non-skilled OSCE Questions

1. **Interpret the lead II ECG shown below.**

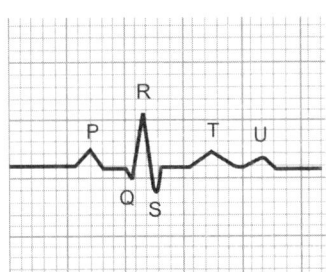

Ans. It is a normal ECG tracings consisting of waveform which indicate electrical events during one heart beat.

These waveforms are P, Q, R, S, T and U waves.
- P wave indicates atrial depolarization.
- QRS complex follows the P wave. The QRS complex represents ventricular depolarization.
- T wave is normally a modest upward waveform, representing ventricular repolarization.
- U wave indicates the recovery of the Purkinje conduction fibers.

2. **Calculate the heart rate from given ECG.**

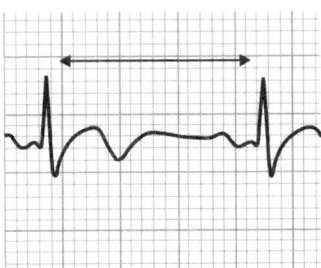

Ans. Count the number of small boxes for a typical RR interval. Divide this number into 1,500 to determine heart rate. In the second image, the number of small boxes for the RR interval is 21.5.

$$\text{Heart rate} = \frac{60 \text{ sec} \times 25 \text{ mm}}{\text{RR interval (mm)}} = \frac{1,500 \text{ (mm)}}{21.5 \text{ mm}}$$

The heart rate is 69.8.

3. **What does PR interval indicate? What is its normal duration? Calculate the PR interval from the given graph.**

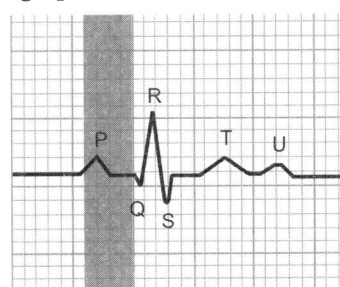

Ans. The PR interval indicates AV conduction time. Normally, this interval is 0.12–0.20 seconds.

There are five small boxes from beginning of P wave, beginning of Q wave: $5 \times 0.04 = 0.2$ seconds.

The PR interval in the above ECG tracing is 0.2 seconds.

4. **What does QRS indicate? Measure the duration of the QRS wave.**

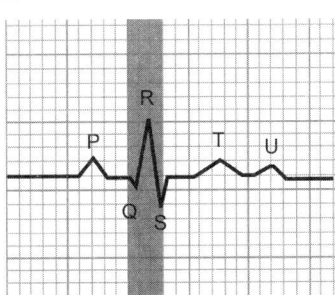

Ans. QRS complex indicates ventricular depolarization. The duration of QRS wave is three small squares: $3 \times 0.04 = 0.12$ seconds.

5. **What does QT interval denote? What is its normal duration? Calculate the QT interval from the given graph.**

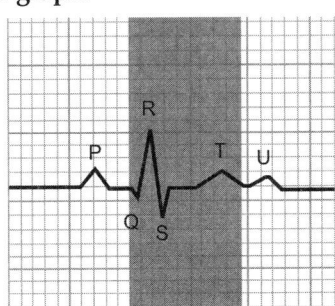

Ans. QT interval denotes ventricular depolarization and ventricular repolarization. Normally QT interval is 0.36–0.44 seconds (9–11 boxes)

The QT interval is 10 small boxes: $10 \times 0.04 = 0.40$ seconds.

VIVA QUESTIONS

1. **What is electrocardiography?**

Ans. Electrocardiography (ECG) is the recording of the electrical changes occurring during the process of depolarization and repolarisation of the heart.

2. **What is the cause of P, QRS and T waves in ECG?**

Ans. P wave is a positive wave, indicating the sum of all the electrical potentials produced during the depolarisation of both atria and the spreading of the electrical activity from SA node throughout the atrial musculature. P wave precedes atrial systole and initiates the atrial contraction.

QRS wave is due to spreading of depolarisation wave through the ventricular muscles, thus initiates ventricular systole (depolarisation). QRS wave precedes isovolumetric contraction.

T wave precedes ventricular diastole and indicates the initiation of ventricular repolarisation (relaxation).

3. **What are the indications for echocardiography in patients?**

Ans. Echocardiography is a non-invasive tool for imaging the heart of the surrounding intra-thoracic structures to diagnose various cardiac diseases to assess cardiac function.

It helps to evaluate size of cardiac chambers, study the thickness and movement of the wall, study the structure and movement of the valves, find out congenital cardiac anomalies, detect pericardial and pleural fluid, identify mass lesions within and adjacent to the heart and diagnose valvular and myocardial pathology.

MULTIPLE CHOICE QUESTIONS

1. **The standard configuration of an ECG recording is:**
   A. 25 mm/sec, 0.5 mV/cm
   B. 25 mm/sec, 1 mV/cm
   C. 50 mm/sec, 0.5 mV/cm
   D. 50 mm/sec, 1 mV/cm

2. **The significance of ECG includes**
   A. It is a non-invasive method to evaluate cardiac function
   B. To diagnose ventricular hypertrophy
   C. To evaluate conduction system blocks, myocardial infarction and drug effects, etc
   D. All of the above

3. **ST elevation suggests**
   A. Myocardial infarction
   B. Heart block
   C. Pan systolic murmur
   D. Marfan's syndrome

4. **What is the common cause of left axis deviation?**
   A. Right ventricular hypertrophy
   B. Atrial septal defects
   C. Ventricular septal defects
   D. Defects of the conduction system

5. **What is the duration of a normal PR-interval?**
   A. 0.04–0.08 seconds (1–2 small squares)
   B. 0.12–2.0 seconds (3–5 small squares)
   C. 0.08–0.12 seconds (2–3 small squares)
   D. 0.23–0.43 seconds (5–11 small squares)

Answers:

1 B	2 D	3 A	4 D	5 B

HISTORICAL ASPECT

Willem Einthoven (1860–1927)

Willem Einthoven was a Dutch physiologist who discovered the procedure for recording the electrical activity of heart and it came to be known as electrocardiography. Einthoven invented a string galvanometer in 1903 and with it developed an improved method for measuring the electrical changes that take place in the body upon the contraction of the heart. Einthoven identified a number of electrical waves associated with a beating heart. He opined that some of these waves result from contractions and electrical changes in the atria and ventricles of the heart. Einthoven assigned the letters P, Q, R, S and T to the various deflections and described the electrocardiographic features of a number of cardiovascular disorders. In 1924, he was awarded the Nobel Prize in Medicine for his discovery.

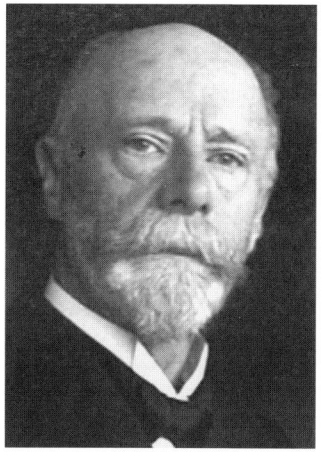

Willem Einthoven

RECENT UPDATES

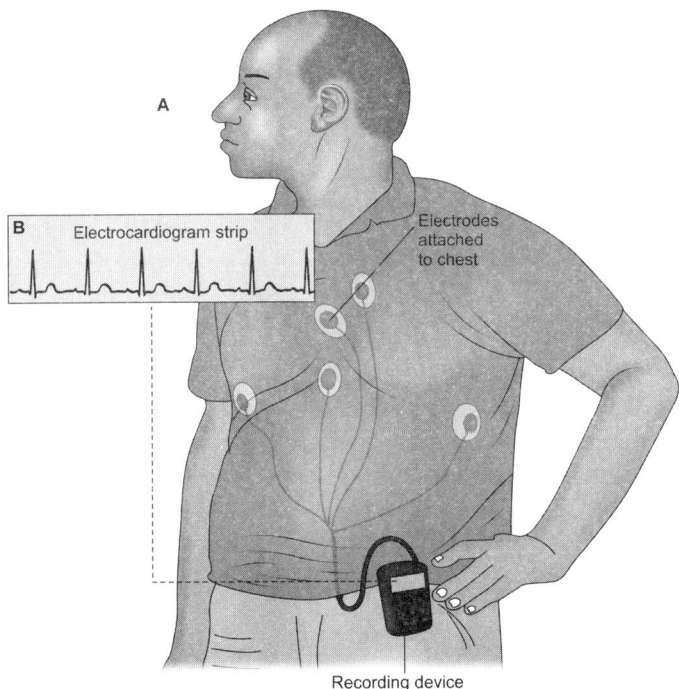

A

B Electrocardiogram strip

Electrodes attached to chest

Recording device

Fig. 17.2 Holter monitor

Holter monitor device continuously records the heart rhythms usually for 24 hours on being tied and applied to the patient. This ambulatory electrocardiograph is battery operated and can be carried in a pocket or a small pouch or worn around the neck or waist. It is connected to electrodes (small conducting patches) which are stuck onto the patient's chest. After 24 hours, the monitor can be viewed by the physician so as to assess patient's symptoms and activities to determine if there have been any irregular heart rhythms.

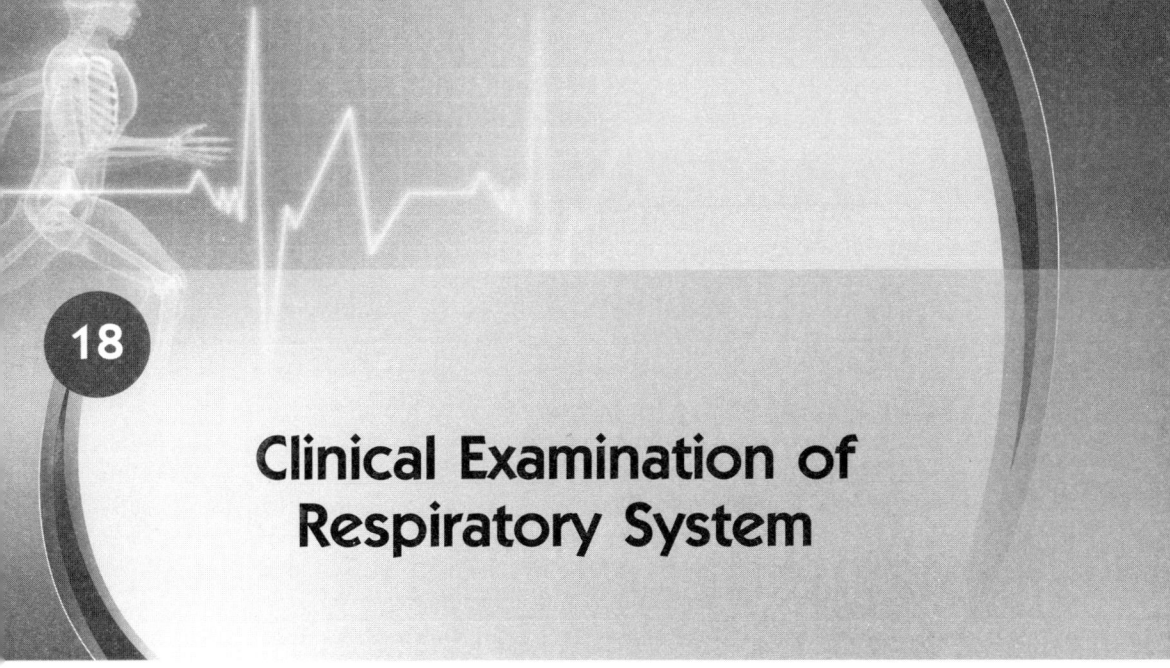

18

Clinical Examination of Respiratory System

Learning Objectives
After learning the practicals, the students should be able to: Understand the importance of findings of inspection, palpation, percussion and auscultation of respiratory system and correlate it with associated respiratory disorders.

INTRODUCTION

The respiratory examination is performed as part of the physical examination or when a patient presents with complaints of cough, breathlessness, chest pain or any history suggestive of lung involvement.

Instruments: Stethoscope, measuring tape and torch.

Method

1. Ask the individual to sit upright on an examination table. Ensure adequate lighting is available in the room.
2. The patient is asked to remove the clothing over the chest.
3. Perform the general clinical examination in the patient/individual noting his/her pulse, body temperature, blood pressure, for the presence of pallor, cyanosis, clubbing, edema and lymphadenopathy.
4. The respiratory examination is carried out in different stages.

Position of the patient: The patient or any individual in whom respiratory system is being examined is asked to sit comfortably on chair or in case of grievous patient may lie supine on examination couch.

Inspection: Inspect the chest from the front, back, along the midaxillary line and over the shoulders and note for:

A. **Shape and deformity of the chest:** The normal chest is bilaterally symmetrical and elliptical in cross section. Observe for any kyphosis (abnormal anterior-posterior curvature of the spine), scoliosis (abnormal lateral curvature of the spine), pectus excavatum (sternum sunken into the chest), pectus carinatum (sternum protruding from the chest) or barrel shape of chest.

B. **Movements of the chest:** Confirm whether the chest movements are equal on both sides and note for frequency and regular rhythm of breathing.

C. **Respiratory rate:** Count the respiratory rate and look for regularity of the rhythm. Holding the patient hand and continuing conversation with patient enquiring his/her health profile, the respiratory moments can be observed and respiratory rate counted. This will not make the patient aware and conscious, otherwise voluntary efforts by patient in nervousness may alter the rate.

D. **Type of respiration:** Note whether the respiration is abdomino-thoracic (seen in men and young children) or thoraco-abdominal (seen in women).

E. **Chest expansion:** Note the degree of the chest expansion and whether it is similar on both sides of the chest.

F. **Position of trachea:** Normally the trachea is central or slightly deviated to the right.

Palpation

1. Palpate and confirm the position of the trachea and the apex beat.

2. Measure the chest expansion using a measuring tape. (Normally, the chest get expanded by 5 cm or more during inspiration.)

3. Compare the chest expansion on both sides. Place the palm of both hands on either side of the chest of the subject and touch the tips of the two thumbs in the midline in front and back of the chest. The subject should be asked to take a deep breath and the distance of displacement of the thumbs from the midline is noted and this indicates the extent of expansion.

4. Vocal fremitus: It refers to vibrations setup by the voice which is conducted from the larynx through the trachea, bronchi and lung tissue to the chest wall. This is detected by placing the hand of the examiner on the chest. The patient/individual are asked to repeat "99" continuously. Place the ulnar border of your palm on corresponding areas on both sides of the subject's chest and compare the vibration set up by the voice. Vocal fremitus is decreased in pleural effusion and increased in consolidation.

Percussion

It is done to compare the degree of resonance over corresponding areas on either sides of the chest. The degree of resonance may differ in different parts of the chest wall. It is most resonant below the scapulae posteriorly and clavicles anteriorly.

Percussion is performed as: Place the middle finger of the left hand (pleximeter) firmly on the part to be percussed and strike the back of its middle phalanx perpendicularly with the tip of the middle finger of your right hand. The percussing finger needs to be bent so that its terminal phalanx is at right angles and it strikes the pleximeter finger exactly perpendicular.

Rules for percussion
1. The stroke should be promptly made by movement at the wrist.
2. The long axis of the pleximeter finger should be parallel to the edge of the organ being percussed.
3. Percussion should be done from more resonant to a less resonant area.

The students should percuss all areas of the chest keeping the pleximeter finger in the intercostal spaces. Ask the subject to keep his/her hand over the head while percussing the sides of the chest. Ask the subject to cross his/her arms in front as you percuss the back of the chest. Lung resonance is impaired in consolidation and fibrosis of the lung. The resonance is stony dull in pleural effusion. Lung resonance is increased in pneumothorax.

Auscultation

Auscultation is to be performed all over the chest and the auscultatory findings of two sides are compared.

The following points are to be noted:

Character of the breath sounds: There are two typical types of breath sounds: (i) vesicular and (ii) bronchial. Vesicular breath sounds are produced by the passage of air in and out of normal lung tissue and are heard all over the chest under normal conditions. The vesicular breathing is low pitched and rustling in character. The inspiratory sound is intense and audible during the whole of inspiration. The expiratory sound follows the inspiration without a distinct pause. The inspiratory sound is heard for a time twice as long as the expiratory sound. Bronchial breath sounds are produced by the passage of air through the trachea and large bronchi. This inspiratory sound is moderately intense and becomes inaudible before the end of inspiration. The expiratory sound is more intense and the duration extends through the greater part of expiration.

Vocal resonance: Auscultate the chest each time the subject repeats "99". Vocal resonance is increased in consolidation and diminished in pleural thickening, effusion and pneumothorax.

Abnormal sounds: These are found in disease states.

Examples:

Wheeze: These are continuous musical sound on expiration or inspiration. A wheeze results of narrowed airways. It is commonly heard in patients of asthma and emphysema.

Rhonchi: They are characterized by low pitched, musical bubbly sounds heard on inspiration and expiration. Rhonchi are heard due to presence of viscous fluid in the airways.

Crackles: This is an intermittent, nonmusical and brief sounds heard during inspiration only. These are the result of sudden opening of alveoli due to increased air pressure during inspiration. This is seen in patients of congestive cardiac failure.

Stridor is a high-pitched musical breath sound resulting from turbulent airflow in the larynx or lower in the bronchial tree. The common causes are typically obstructive such as foreign body in airway.

DENTAL IMPLICATION

As a dental practitioner the knowledge of respiratory disorders and the clinical signs and symptoms associated with them helps for better evaluation, screening and management of patients of respiratory disorders reporting to dental clinic with dental disorders. The review with physician prior to dental procedures or surgery is recommended for effective management and recovery of patient.

OBJECTIVE STRUCTURED CLINICAL EXAMINATION (OSCE) QUESTIONS

1. Describe the various types of shapes of the chest.

Ans. The variation in chest shape types are kyphosis (abnormal anterior-posterior curvature of the spine), scoliosis (abnormal lateral curvature of the spine), pectus excavatum (sternum sunken into the chest), pectus carinatum (sternum protruding from the chest) and barrel shape of chest.

2. Describe the method for counting the respiratory rate.

Ans. The respiratory rate is an observational evaluation and should be meticulously calculated by carefully observing the moments of the chest.

VIVA QUESTIONS

1. Explain the physiological basis of compliance.

Ans. The slope of the pressure–volume curve, i.e. the change in volume per unit pressure is known as *compliance*. The compliance in case of the human lung is 0.15 L/cm H_2O.

Compliance is reduced when
1. The pulmonary venous pressure is increased and the lung becomes engorged with blood.
2. Diseases causing fibrosis of the lung, e.g. chronic restrictive lung disease
3. The lung remains unventilated for a while as in atelectasis and
4. In alveolar oedema due to insufficiency of alveolar inflation

In chronic obstructive pulmonary disease (COPD, e.g. emphysema), the alveolar walls progressively degenerates and increases the compliance.

2. Define anatomical dead space.

Ans. It is the volume of the conducting airways. It is approximately 150 mL.

3. Define forced expiratory volume (FEV).

Ans. It is the volume of gas exhaled in one second by a forceful expiration following a full inspiration (FEV1). The total volume of the gas exhaled after a complete and full inspiration represents the vital capacity. However, this value may be slightly smaller than the vital capacity measured with slow (normal speed) expiration. Therefore, this value is called *forced vital capacity* (FVC). The normal ratio of the FEV1 is 80% of that of forced vital capacity.

4. Define forced expiratory flow (FEF 25–75).

Ans. This measurement represents the expiratory flow rate over the middle half of the FVC (between 25 and 75%); obtained by identifying the 25% and 75% volume points of FVC, measuring the time between these points and therewith calculating the flow rate.

5. Discuss the criterion of classifying lung diseases as restrictive or obstructive disorder.

Ans. The lung diseases can be classified as restrictive or obstructive. In restrictive lung diseases the vital capacity is reduced to below normal levels; however, the rate at which the vital capacity is forcefully exhaled is normal. In obstructive lung disease the vital capacity is normal because lung tissue is not damage and its compliance is unchanged but the increased airway resistance makes expiration more difficult and takes longer time. Obstructive disorders are therefore diagnosed by tests that measure the rate of forced expiration. A significant decrease in FEV1 and FEF 25–75% suggests an obstructive lung disease.

MULTIPLE CHOICE QUESTIONS

1. Which of the following is inactivated in the lung?
   A. Angiotensin II
   B. Angiotensin I
   C. Oestrogen
   D. Bradykinin

2. The partial pressure of oxygen in dry air at sea level:
   A. 153 mmHg
   B. 119 mmHg
   C. 159 mmHg
   D. 100 mmHg

3. Type II pneumocytes
   A. Develop from type I pneumocytes
   B. Secret calcium
   C. Are very flat and practically devoid of organelles
   D. Metabolise surfactant

4. Factors that favor formation of carbaminohemoglobin include:
   A. Carbonic anhydrase
   B. Sodium bicarbonate
   C. Aluminium hydroxide
   D. None of the above

5. **For a normal Hb-O$_2$ dissociation curve, the most correct relationship is:**
   A. PaO$_2$ 60 mmHg, SaO$_2$ 91%
   B. PaO$_2$ 132 mmHg, SaO$_2$ 98%
   C. PaO$_2$ 68 mmHg, SaO$_2$ 97%
   D. PaO$_2$ 340 mmHg, SaO$_2$ 99%

Answers:

1 D	2 C	3 D	4 D	5 D

HISTORICAL ASPECT

Michael Servetus (1553)

The first description of the function of pulmonary circulation was made by Ibn al-Nafis in the year 1242 in Egypt but later more relevant details regarding it was stated by Michael Servetus (1553) and William Harvey (1616).

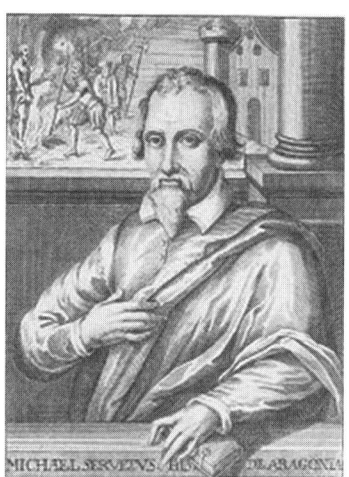

Michael Servetus

He decided to return to the study of medicine and he was a medical student from 1536–38 at the University of Paris. He followed the well-known anatomist Andreas Vesalius as assistant to Hans Gunther in dissection practical studies. Gunther wrote that "Michael Villonovanus" had perfect knowledge of Galen's work. Servetus later came to differ from Galen in the understanding of pulmonary circulation. Galen had supposed that the aeration of the blood takes place in the heart and lungs as a fairly minor function. Servetus concluded from his experimentation that the transformation of the blood accomplished by the release of waste gases and the infusion of air occurred in the lungs.

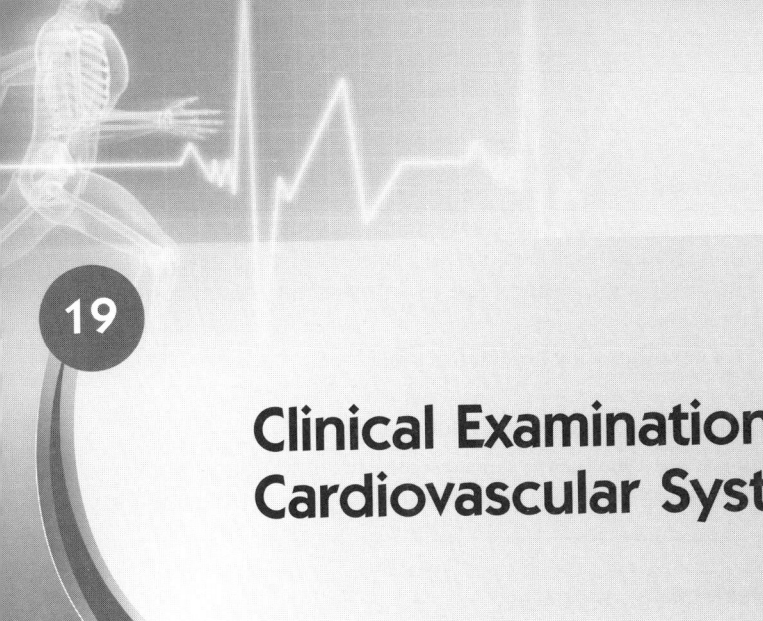

19

Clinical Examination of Cardiovascular System

INTRODUCTION

The precordial examination is also called the cardiac examination. It is carried out as part of a physical examination or when a patient presents with complaints of chest pain, associated breathlessness, palpitation, restlessness, sweating or any signs and symptoms suggestive of a cardiovascular pathology.

Instruments: Stethoscope, sphygmomanometer, measuring tape and torch.

PROCEDURES

1. Ask the individual to sit upright on an examination table. Ensure adequate lighting is available in the room.
2. The patient is asked to remove the clothing over the chest.
3. Perform the general clinical examination in the patient/individual noting his/her pulse, body temperature, blood pressure, for the presence of pallor, cyanosis, clubbing, edema and lymphadenopathy.

   The cardiovascular examination is carried out under the following headings:
   - Inspection
   - Palpation
   - Percussion
   - Auscultation

Inspection

The cardiovascular examination should be carried out positioning the patient the supine position tilted up at 45°. The neck should be made prominent for visualization of pulsation.

1. Inspect the patient status for whether they are comfortable at rest or obviously short of breath.
2. Identify the shape of the chest and observe its bilateral symmetery.
3. If any prominent veins visible on the chest wall, these are prominently seen in case of intrathoracic growth, secondary to portal obstruction and obstruction to inferior vena cava.
4. Position of the trachea.
5. Presence of any precordial bulge or depression.
6. Position of apical pulsation, if visible.
7. Inspect the neck for increased jugular venous pressure (JVP) or abnormal waves. The JVP is increased in pregnancy (as a result of increased circulating blood volume), right heart failure, atrial myxoma and in obstruction to superior vena cava. The jugular veins communicate directly with the right atrium. Therefore, the fluctuations in right atrial pressure during the cardiac cycle generate a pulse which is transmitted backward into the jugular veins.

Palpation

1. The position of the trachea is to be confirmed by palpation for the trachea in the suprasternal notch and note if it is central or deviated to one side.
2. Confirm and note the position and character of the apex beat. Place the palm of the right hand over the apex, localize the apex beat by using the medial border of the palm and then feel it with the tips of the fingers. The apex beat is defined as the lowermost and outermost definite palpable cardiac impulse usually felt in the fifth left intercostal space, 1 cm medial to the midclavicular line.
3. Place the hypothenar eminence of your right palm on the left mid and lower parasternal region of the patient/individual and confirm if parasternal heave is present.
4. Palpate the precordium for presence of a thrill (a palpable murmur which resembles the purring of a cat).

Percussion

The rules of percussion are:
1. The stroke should be promptly made by movement at the wrist.
2. The long axis of the pleximeter finger should be parallel to the edge of the organ being percussed.
3. Percussion should be done from more resonant to a less resonant area.

Percuss lightly from the sides toward the heart in order to define the cardiac dullness, and to delineate the borders of the heart.

Auscultation

Auscultate the precordium in the following areas using a stethoscope:

- **Mitral area** corresponds to the region of the apex beat.

- **Tricuspid area** is present to the left of the lower end of the sternum.

- **Aortic area** is present to the right of the sternum, in the second intercostal space.

- **Pulmonary area** is present to the left of the sternum in the second intercostal space.

  In each of the above four areas note the character of the first and second heart sounds which can be differentiated by their pitch and duration.

  Palpate the left common carotid artery in the neck while auscultating for the heart sounds.

  The students should note the reasons for the four heart sounds (S1, S2, S3 and S4).

Heart sound	Occurs during	Associated with
S1	Isovolumetric contraction	Closure of mitral and tricuspid valves
S2	Isovolumetric relaxation	Closure of aortic and pulmonic valves
S3	Early ventricular filling	Normal in children; in adults, associated with ventricular dilation (e.g. ventricular systolic failure)
S4	Atrial contraction	Associated with stiff, low compliant ventricle (e.g. ventricular hypertrophy)

DENTAL IMPLICATION

As a dental practitioner, the knowledge of cardiovascular disorders and the clinical signs and symptoms associated with them helps for better evaluation, screening and management of patients of respiratory disorders reporting to dental clinic with dental disorders. The review with physician prior to dental procedures or surgery is recommended for effective management and recovery of patient.

OBJECTIVE STRUCTURED CLINICAL EXAMINATION (OSCE) QUESTIONS

1. **Enlist the clinical conditions in whom JVP is raised.**

Ans. The causes of raised JVP are:
   1. Pericardial effusion/pulmonary embolism/pericardial constriction
   2. Quantity of fluid increased (iatrogenic fluid overload)
   3. Right heart failure or congestive heart failure
   4. Superior vena caval obstruction
   5. Tricuspid regurgitation/tricuspid stenosis/tamponade (cardiac)

2. **Discuss the procedure of palpation of apex beat.**

Ans. Apex beat: The patient may be asked to lie down on examination couch and later asked to lie at left lateral decubitus position. Place the palm of the right hand over the apex, localize the apex beat by using the medial border of the palm and then feel it with the tips of the fingers. The apex beat is usually felt in the fifth left intercostal space, 1 cm medial to the midclavicular line.

3. **Locate the position over chest where the first and second heart sound are better heard.**

Ans. The first heart sound is better heard in apex along the mitral and also at tricuspid area. The second heart sound is best heard in pulmonary and aortic areas.

VIVA QUESTIONS

1. **Name the pacemaker of the heart.**

Ans. The SA node is the pacemaker of heart as physiologically it controls the heart rate.

2. **Describe the heart valves.**

Ans. Heart consists of four valves
   - Two atrioventricular (AV) valves between atria and ventricles
   - Aortic and pulmonary valves at junction of ventricles and great arteries.

3. **Discuss the functions of heart.**

Ans. The function of the heart is to generate blood pressure so as to produce a gradient that pushes blood through the vascular system. The heart works in conjunction with cardiovascular centres and peripheral blood vessels to achieve this goal. It regulates blood supply by the sympathetic and parasympathetic control by cardiovascular centre in CNS to alter the contraction rate and force to match blood delivery to meet the metabolic needs. The pulmonary circuit takes blood to and from the lungs and systemic circuit vessels transport blood to and from body tissues.

4. **Define cardiac cycle.**

Ans. Cardiac cycle is the sequence of events of pressure and volume changes, and changes of the electrical potential during the period between two successive ventricular contractions.

5. **What are the causes for first and second heart sound?**

Ans. The first heart sound is due to the closure of AV valves which occur during ventricular systole. The second heart sound is due to the closure of the aortic and pulmonary valves at protodiastole phase of the cardiac cycle.

6. **Enlist the factors which affect blood pressure.**

Ans. The factors which affect blood pressure are:
   - Cardiac output
   - Total blood volume
   - Blood viscosity

• Elasticity of arteries
• Resistance (vessel lumen size and smoothness)

7. **What is baroreceptor reflex?**

Ans. The arterial blood pressure is reflex controlled by pressure sensitive nerve endings known as *baroreceptors; located in the* carotid bodies and along aortic arch; which are sensitive to stretch of the arterial wall. Baroreceptors send afferent impulses through sinus and aortic nerves (buffer nerves) to vasomotor areas of the central nervous system which monitor beat to beat changes in arterial pressure. The central nervous system as reflex response alters cardiac output by the sympathetic and parasympathetic divisions of autonomic nervous system which alter the vascular resistance by vasoconstriction or vasodilatation.

8. **Discuss the long term effect of exercise on heart.**

Ans. The long term effects of exercise on heart are: Aerobic exercise strengthens the heart, the walls become thicker and stronger, the stroke volume increases and the heart becomes a more efficient pump. Training also results in new capillaries growing to improve the supply of blood to the muscles.

9. **Describe the tests for cardiovascular fitness.**

Ans. The tests for cardiovascular fitness are:

• The best way of measuring cardiovascular fitness is to calculate a performer's **VO$_2$ max.** This measures the maximum amount of oxygen the body can take in.

   However, calculating VO$_2$ max requires very specialized equipment.

• An alternative is the **bleep test**. Performers have to do 20 metre shuttle runs, keeping pace with a series of recorded bleeps which gradually get faster. The point at which the performer has to drop out is recorded.

• The easiest test is the **12-minute run**. Performers simply run for 12 minutes and the distance covered is recorded.

• Testing speed, flexibility and balance

   Speed is easy to test. Simply record how fast a performer can sprint a short distance. 100 metres and 60 metres distances are often used.

   Flexibility can be tested by measuring a performer's range of movement. A common test for flexibility is the **sit and reach test.**

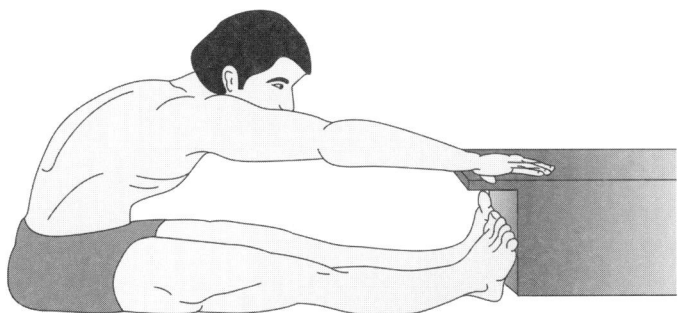

Exhibit 19.1 Testing speed, flexibility and balance

How far the performer can reach relative to their feet is measured on a ruler.

Balance can be tested using the **stork stand test**. The performer stands on one leg, with their free foot on their standing knee. How long they can hold the position for is timed.

Agility can be tested by setting up an **agility run** and timing how long it takes for a performer to complete it.

When **retesting** performers to measure improvement, you must take care that the agility run is set up exactly the same as before.

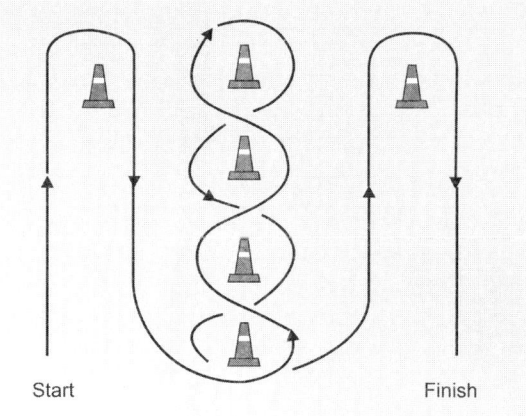

Start   Finish

Exhibit 19.2 Agility test

Muscular endurance can be tested easily by seeing how many times a performer can repeat a movement requiring strength. **Sit-ups** and **press-ups** are often used.

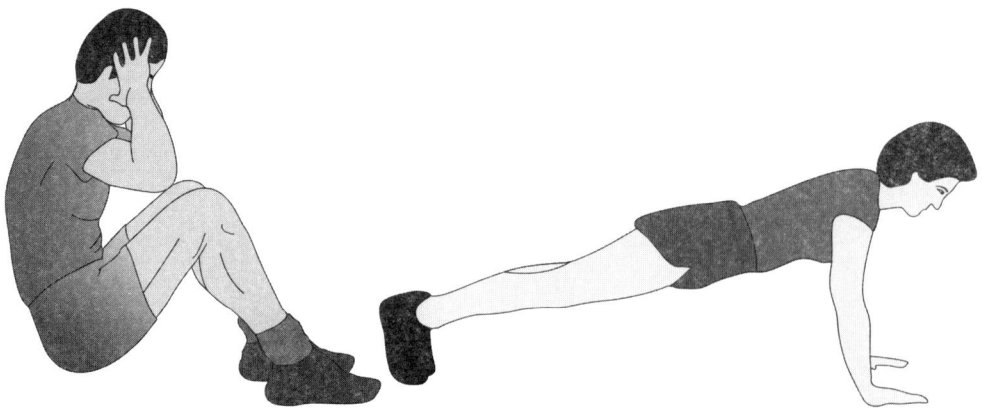

Exhibit 19.3 Sit-ups and press-ups

MULTIPLE CHOICE QUESTIONS

1. **In a normal cardiac cycle (same as CV01 but we remembered the options as):**
   A. RA ejection precedes LA ejection
   B. RV contraction starts before LV contraction
   C. LV ejection starts before RV ejection
   D. Pulmonary valve closes before aortic valve

2. **In a normal heart at rest the LV end-systolic volume is:**
   A. 10 to 30 mL
   B. 50 to 70 mL
   C. 120 to 150 mL
   D. 80 to 100 mL

3. **Which one of the following (does/does not) cause (an increased/a decreased) heart rate?**
   A. Bainbridge reflex
   B. Carotid chemoreflex
   C. Bezold-Jarisch reflex
   D. Hering-Breuer reflex

4. **The highest oxygen extraction is found in the:**
   A. Carotid body
   B. Heart
   C. Kidney
   D. Brain

5. **Coronary blood flow is:**
   A. Dominant in left coronary artery in 60% of people
   B. Better supply to subendocardium in systole
   C. Better supply to subendocardium in diastole
   D. Better supply to left ventricle in systole

6. **Baroreceptors located in all except:**
   A. Carotid sinus
   B. Carotid body
   C. Right atrium
   D. Aortic arch

Answers:

1 A	2 B	3 D	4 B	5 C	6 B

HISTORICAL ASPECTS

Leonardo da Vinci (1452–1519)

He investigated and studied the coronary arteries. William Harvey (1578–1657) Physician to King Charles I is credited with discovering circulatory mechanism of heart. Harvey understanding of the relationship between arteries and veins was existence of a unified circulatory system. Friedrich Hoffmann (1660–1742) was a chief professor of cardiology at the University of Halle and found that coronary heart disease emerged in the "reduced passage of the blood within the coronary arteries". He described the heart as a muscle, understood the role of the coronary vessels and was the first to mention the moderator band and the relation of the systole to the pulse. He also discovered the hemodynamic function of the sinuses of Valsalva in the

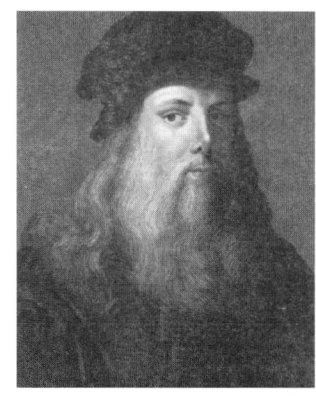

Leonardo da Vinci

closure mechanism of the aortic valve. Leonardo's notes and drawings on the heart are a fine example of his open mind and keen observation.

Coronary Diseases

William Osler (1849–1919), a cardiologist was first to explain angina and opined that it is a syndrome rather than a disease in itself.

In 1912, **James B. Herrick (1861–1954),** the American cardiologist discovered that the gradual narrowing of the coronary arteries could be the cause of angina. He invented the term "heart attack".

John Gofman (1918–2007), in the year 1950, as a researcher along with his associates at University of California identified today's low-density lipoprotein (LDL) and high-density lipoprotein (HDL). He found out that patient who developed atherosclerosis had elevated levels of LDL and low levels of HDL.

Ancel Keys (1904–2004), an American scientist, in the year 1950 discovered that heart disease was rare in some Mediterranean populations who consumed a lower fat diet. He also observed that the Japanese had low-fat diets and low rates of heart disease as support to his theory of that fat was the cause of heart disease.

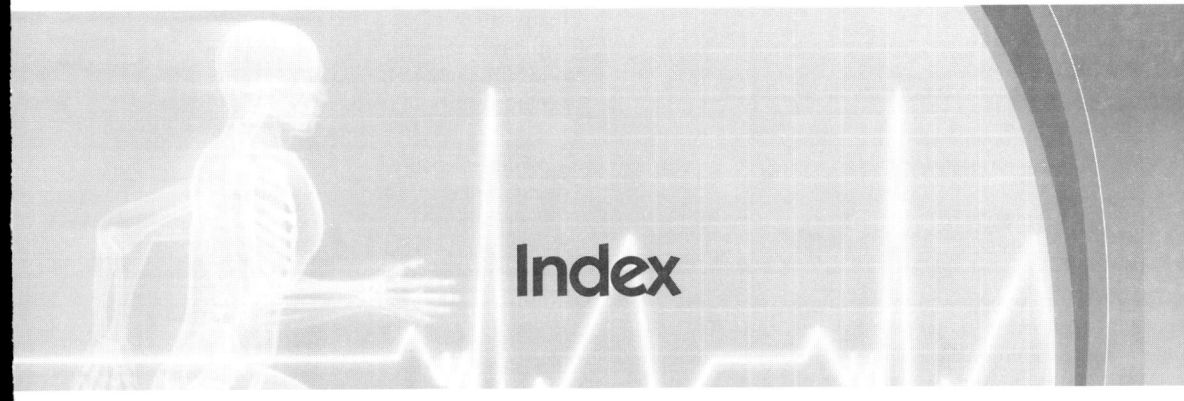

Index